"The Hour of Eugenics"

"*The Hour of Eugenics*"

RACE, GENDER, AND NATION IN LATIN AMERICA

Nancy Leys Stepan

Cornell University Press

ITHACA AND LONDON

First published 1991 by Cornell University Press
First printing, Cornell Paperbacks, 1996

Printed in the United States of America

Library of Congress Cataloging-in-Publication Data

Stepan, Nancy.
   The hour of eugenics : race, gender, and nation in Latin America /
Nancy Leys Stepan.
       p.   cm.
   Includes index.
   ISBN 0–8014–2569–7 (alk. paper). — ISBN 0–8014–9795–7 (pbk. :
alk. paper)
     1. Eugenics—Latin America.   I. Title.
   HQ755.5.L29S74   1991
   363.9'2'098—dc20   91–55051

Cloth printing   10 9 8 7 6 5 4 3 2 1
Paperback printing   10 9 8 7 6 5 4

Contents

Acknowledgments

Many people have helped me with this book by commenting on the manuscript, sharing ideas and references, talking about common research interests, or taking the trouble to drive me to out-of-the-way libraries. In retrospect it is often difficult to say exactly how what each one said or did made a difference, but I know that it did. I list these friends and colleagues in alphabetical order and thank them all for contributing in ways direct and indirect: Mark B. Adams, Marcos Cueto, Geraldo Forbes, Jean Franco, Sander L. Gilman, Thomas F. Glick, Ruth Leys, Larissa Lomnitz, Mary Nash, Julyan Peard, Paulo Sergio Pinheiro, Carole Satyamurti, William E. Schneider, Thomas E. Skidmore, Ann Laura Stoler, Sheila Faith Weiss, and Eduardo Zimmerman. At Columbia University students in my seminars have often contributed to my thinking, as have colleagues involved in workshops and meetings at the Institute for Research on Women and Gender.

This book is based on research carried out during several visits to Brazil, Argentina, and Mexico, where I consulted materials in various national, historical, medical, and agricultural libraries. The libraries of the Faculty of Medicine in Buenos Aires and the Oswaldo Cruz Institute in Rio de Janeiro were particularly fruitful for my project. I also relied on collections in the National Academy of Medicine, the New York Public Library, and the Health Sciences Library of Columbia University in New York, as well as the National

Library of Medicine in Washington. In London I had the pleasure of working at the Wellcome Institute for the History of Medicine. I am very grateful to the many librarians who assisted me in all these places. Work on this book was greatly assisted by a Guggenheim Fellowship in 1986–1987 and by a grant from the National Science Foundation's Program in the History and Philosophy of Science and Technology (summer 1986 and 1987). A stint as a Senior Fellow at the Society for the Humanities, Cornell University, in the fall of 1987 provided excellent working conditions and lively discussions. My thanks also go to the members of the Institute for Advanced Studies, University of São Paulo, for the invitation to exchange ideas with Brazilian scholars. I also record my very good fortune in working with John G. Ackerman, Kay Scheuer, and Marilyn M. Sale at Cornell University Press; they have all been exemplary in their attention and editorial help.

I thank Oxford University Press for permission to reprint portions of a chapter that appeared in *The Wellborn Science: Eugenics in Germany, France, Brazil, and Russia*, ed. Mark B. Adams (New York, 1990), and the American Philosophical Society in Philadelphia for permission to quote from the Davenport papers held in its collections.

Lastly, it is to my husband, Alfred Stepan, that I can truly say I owe the most. His intellectual drive, zest for life and adventure, and unfailing good humor make all the difference, and this book is dedicated to him.

NANCY LEYS STEPAN

New York City

"The Hour of Eugenics"

Introduction: Science
and Social Knowledge

This book addresses the scientific and social movement known as eugenics, a word invented in 1883 (from the Greek *eugenēs*, meaning "wellborn") by the British scientist Francis Galton to encompass the social uses to which knowledge of heredity could be put in order to achieve the goal of "better breeding."[1] Others defined eugenics as a movement to "improve" the human race or, indeed, to preserve the "purity" of particular groups. As a science, eugenics was based on supposedly new understanding of the laws of human heredity. As a social movement, it involved proposals that society ensure the constant improvement of its hereditary makeup by encouraging "fit" individuals and groups to reproduce themselves and, perhaps more

---

1. It was the U.S. eugenist Charles B. Davenport who gave this succinct definition in his book *Heredity in Relation to Eugenics* (New York: Henry Holt, 1911), p. 1. *Please note*: Throughout this book I have chosen to refer to the people pursuing eugenics as "eugenists." This usage is contrary to current fashion (in which "eugenicists" is preferred) but historically one of the possible appellations, and the one normally used in British eugenics before World War II. That eugenics originated as an idea in Britain is one reason for prefering the term.

Portuguese spelling: Portuguese spelling and accenting have undergone several changes in the course of the twentieth century. I have used modern spellings and diacritical marks for people's names in the text but have retained the original orthography in the citations, in the belief that this practice would aid other historians. Unless otherwise indicated, translations are my own.

important, by discouraging or preventing the "unfit" from contributing their unfitness to future generations.

Practically speaking, eugenics encouraged the scientific and "rational" management of the hereditary makeup of the human species. It also introduced new social ideas and innovative policies of potentially explosive social force—such as the deliberate social selection against supposedly "unfit" individuals, including involuntary surgical sterilization and genetic racism.

The historical significance of eugenics, as well as the possible relevance of eugenics to current developments in human genetics and reproduction, has stimulated a surge of interest in the eugenics of the interwar years. This said, however, it is still surprising how restricted the study of eugenics is, especially when we consider the quasi-international currency of eugenics between the two world wars and its connections to many of the large themes of modern history, such as nationalism, racism, sexuality and gender, social hygiene, and the development of modern genetics itself. Eugenics societies, organizations, pressure groups, and legislation appeared in countries as different from one another as England, Italy, France, Japan, the Soviet Union, Sweden, Peru, and Australia, yet new studies of eugenics hardly reflect this fact. Recent work focuses largely on Britain and the United States, with even Germany, where eugenics reached its apogee of extremity and nastiness in National Socialism, coming a distant third.

"Latin" areas (the term used by the Latin International Federation of Eugenics Societies, founded in 1935, to refer to Italy, France, and Belgium as well as Latin American countries) are usually ignored, especially Latin America. Yet not only was Latin America oriented to Western science and medicine, and very receptive to European values and ideas; it was the only "third world" and yet postcolonial region where eugenics was taken up in a more or less systematic way. I argue in this book that Latin America is significant precisely because it challenges the more common understanding based on what Daniel Kevles has characterized as the "mainline" eugenics movements of Europe and the United States.[2] The inclusion of Latin American cases—and, more generally, the European Latin countries

2. See Daniel J. Kevles, *In the Name of Eugenics: Genetics and the Uses of Human Heredity* (New York: Knopf, 1985), chap. 6. This is one of the fullest and best accounts of eugenics in Britain and the United States.

with which the region associated itself in eugenics—gives us an expanded sense of the parameters of eugenics and goes a long way, I believe, to explain the extraordinary appeal of a scientific reform movement that after World War II was found to be morally and scientifically unacceptable.

The historical neglect of eugenics in Latin America is, of course, part of the larger neglect of the history of intellectual and cultural life in an area generally presented as being either out of the mainstream or only dimly reflecting European thought. The European bias of the history of ideas is well known, but it is especially strong in science. Latin America is often ignored altogether or it is treated as a consumer and not as a contributor of ideas, and a fairly passive one at that. The implicit assumption is that intellectual historians of Latin America are studying only an attempt to imitate or reproduce a European activity in an alien or unscientific setting. The intellectual gaze always moves from a center outward, toward a problematic periphery.

What historians often fail to appreciate is the contribution a region such as Latin America can make to our knowledge of how ideas become part of the complex fabric of social and political life; historians give too little weight to the construction of intellectual and scientific traditions within the region or to the way these traditions shape the meaning given to ideas, as subjects of interest in their own right. The varied processes of selection and reassemblage of ideas and practices, of their creative elaboration and modification, undertaken by specific groups of people in specific institutional, political, and cultural locations, are left out of consideration. Rarely is the case made that studying an aspect of modern culture in such an area as Latin America may actually change how we understand the meaning of ideas in general; or that Latin American intellectual history may make a difference in how we define a major set of ideas such as Darwinism or what is to count *as* Darwinism—or more generally, as Thomas F. Glick has said, what is to count as normative in intellectual or scientific history.[3]

In this book I argue precisely this point, namely that when we

3. See Glick's discussion in "Reception Studies since 1974," in *The Comparative Reception of Darwinism*, ed. Thomas F. Glick (Chicago: University of Chicago Press, 1988), pp. xi–xxviii; and his observations in "Cultural Issues in the Reception of Relativity," in *The Comparative Reception of Relativity*, ed. Thomas F. Glick (Boston: D. Reidel, 1987), pp. 381–400.

study the history of eugenics in Latin America, as a special kind of social knowledge produced out of, and shaped by, the political, historical, and cultural variables peculiar to the area, our understanding of the meaning of eugenics in general is altered.[4] The terminology of "center" and "periphery" loses much of its analytical force. The book, then, turns what is an implicit convention of intellectual and cultural history on its head by proposing that careful consideration of at least one aspect of the history of ideas and its associated social practices in Latin America will suggest new ways of conceptualizing the meaning of eugenics in the modern era. Eugenics was not unitary and could not be appropriated wholesale. The study of eugenics in Latin America reveals some of the contradictory impulses within the movement and the diverse ways it could be taken up.

The "Normality" of Eugenics

Many people have only a very vague recollection of the word "eugenics" and are often hard put to say what exactly it means. An idea and a movement that once had considerable resonance in the world have almost disappeared from public view. There are good historical and moral reasons for this disappearance, the main one being the link between eugenics and the ghastly acts of the Nazis, who forcibly sterilized hundreds of thousands of people (1 percent of Germany's population) "in the name of eugenics."[5] Another feature of Nazi eugenics is what Robert Jay Lifton, in his powerful and disturbing account of the Nazi doctors, refers to as the "malignant blending of biomedical and politico-racial ideologies."[6] After World War II Nazi eugenics was rightly condemned as a gross perversion of science and morality; the word itself was purged from the vocabulary of science and public debate.

Yet equating eugenics with fascist Germany is problematic on two counts. First, it conceals crucial continuities in eugenics be-

4. Everett Mendelsohn, in "The Social Construction of Scientific Knowledge," remarks that "scientific knowledge is [therefore] fundamentally social knowledge"; see *The Social Production of Scientific Knowledge*, ed. E. Mendelsohn, P. Weingart, and R. Whitley (Boston: D. Reidel, 1977), p. 4.
5. The phrase comes from the title of Kevles's *In the Name of Eugenics* [note 2].
6. Robert Jay Lifton, *The Nazi Doctors: Medical Killing and the Psychology of Genocide* (New York: Basic Books, 1986), p. 274.

tween the fascist and prefascist periods.[7] Second, it tempts historians to avoid discussing the involvement of many other nations in the eugenic experiment. Intellectual practice further aids such avoidance. Historians of science, especially, have a strong tendency to dismiss ideas that later seem obviously biased or hopelessly out of date as "pseudoscientific." Calling eugenics pseudoscientific is a convenient way to set aside the involvement of many prominent scientists in its making and to ignore difficult questions about the political nature of much of the biological and human sciences.

In fact, one of the puzzles about eugenics is that, far from viewing it as a bizarre notion of extremists at the fringes of respectable science and social reform, many well-placed scientists, medical doctors, and social activists endorsed it as an appropriate outcome of developments in the science of human heredity. The success of the First International Eugenics Congress, held in London in 1912, suggested the potentially wide appeal of eugenics, with some 750 participants from several European countries as well as the United States. Two further international eugenics congresses followed in 1921 and 1932 (both in New York). An International Federation of Eugenic Societies was founded in 1921 to coordinate the activities of the numerous national organizations and the various legal initiatives developed since 1912. Eugenics had become so much a part of health reform by the 1920s that a whole discursive field had been, in effect, "eugenicized." Eugenics had its critics, and many of its more extreme social goals and legislative ambitions failed to be met; yet the notion that human individuals and groups varied in their hereditary value and that one day, if not immediately, social policies should be based on these differences was widely accepted in many countries as fundamentally correct.

In recent years, an appreciation of the ubiquity and even the "normality" of eugenic themes and practices between the two world

7. Recent works on German eugenics, before and during the Nazi period, include Paul Weindling, *Health, Race, and German Politics between National Unification and Nazism, 1870–1945* (Cambridge: Cambridge University Press, 1989); Robert N. Proctor, *Racial Hygiene: Medicine under the Nazis* (Cambridge: Harvard University Press, 1988); Sheila Faith Weiss, "The Race Hygiene Movement in Germany," *Osiris* 2d ser. 3 (1987): 193–236, and *Race Hygiene and National Efficiency: The Eugenics of Wilhelm Schallmayer* (Berkeley: University of California Press, 1987); and Peter Weingart, "The Rationalization of Sexual Behavior: The Institutionalization of Eugenics in Germany," *Journal of the History of Biology* 20 (1987): 159–93, and his "German Eugenics between Science and Politics," *Osiris* 2d ser. 5 (1989): 260–82.

wars has led historians to reevaluate eugenics as a social and scientific movement. We are beginning to write the history of eugenics prospectively rather than retrospectively, from the beginning forward, rather than from the end backward. In some respects it may be more important to study eugenics in its non-Nazi forms, because Nazi eugenics was so brutal, so excessive, and so terrifying that it is tempting to view it as a historical aberration. We need to recapture "ordinary" eugenics and its social meanings. What made scientists give their support to ideas and practices that later would seem not only scientifically unsupportable but immoral? Why were over seventy thousand individuals in the United States sterilized involuntarily for eugenic purposes? How did the ordinary eugenics of the 1920s and early 1930s become the extraordinary eugenics of Nazi Germany?[8]

As a topic of study, eugenics offers the historian an opportunity to examine the relationships between science and social life—how social life structures or influences actual developments in hereditarian science, and the uses to which hereditarian science may be put. Eugenics has the further advantage of being contemporary and yet historical: contemporary in that the problems of erecting social policies on the basis of new knowledge in the field of human genetics and reproductive technology are especially pressing today, yet historical in the sense that the eugenics of the pre-1945 period can be viewed as a relatively closed phenomenon of the past on which we can gain some perspective.[9]

Here the study of Latin American eugenics acquires its significance. As I have already stated, even our best studies make no mention of Latin America.[10] This omission would matter little if we

8. Recent works on American and/or British eugenics include Kevles, *In the Name of Eugenics* [note 2]; G. R. Searle, *Eugenics and Politics in Britain* (Leyden: Woordhoff, 1976); Donald A. McKenzie, *Statistics in Britain, 1865–1930: The Social Construction of Scientific Knowledge* (Edinburgh: Edinburgh University Press, 1981); Greta Jones, *Social Hygiene in Twentieth-Century Britain* (London: Croom Helm, 1986).

9. Some people argue that current reproductive technologies and knowledge about genetics involve implicit eugenic issues and decisions that link the present to the past; others maintain that social and policy issues are difficult but not related to eugenics—that is, they do not involve differential breeding of human populations to improve overall genetic fitness.

10. Other Latin countries whose eugenics movements show a family likeness to the Latin American are France, Spain, and Italy. French eugenics, which has an important bearing on Latin American eugenics, has been analyzed recently by William H. Schneider in *Quality and Quantity: The Quest for Biological Regeneration in*

were assured that eugenics always had the same meaning wherever it was found. But meaning, in science as in any other facet of intellectual and cultural life, is never stable. Instead of using prior definitions to exclude novel examples from eugenics, we should extend our historical accounts and, in so doing, probe more deeply the significance of eugenics to modern history. As a region, Latin America is especially rewarding for the analysis of the kinds of themes I have outlined. It was Western in outlook and orientation, yet not merely an imitation of Europe; American, but not North American; "third world" in its poverty, inequality, and dependency but not uniformly poor and similarly dependent across the spectrum of Latin American countries; ethnically and culturally complex, and the site of troubling racist ideologies; culturally Catholic and deeply shaped by traditional gender ideologies, yet not immune to the pull of secularism and modernity. Then, too, the region was involved in nationalist self-making, in which the setting of boundaries between self and other and the creation of identities were increasingly carried out by and through scientific and medical discourses.[11]

Twentieth-Century France (New York: Cambridge University Press, 1990); see also his chapter in *The Wellborn Science: Eugenics in Germany, France, Brazil, and Russia*, ed. Mark B. Adams (New York: Oxford University Press, 1990), pp. 69–109. The French historian Jacques Léonard has contributed some useful articles: see "Le Premier Congrès International d'Eugénique (Londres, 1912) et ses conséquences françaises," *Histoire de Sciences Médicales* 17 (1983): 141–46, and "Eugénisme et Darwinisme: Espoirs et perplexités chez des médecins français du XIXe siècle et du début du XXe siècle," in *De Darwin au Darwinisme: Science et idéologie*, ed. Y. Conry (Paris: Vrin, 1983), pp. 187–207. On Spanish eugenics, see Raquel Alverez Paláez, "Introducción al estudio de la eugenesia española (1900–1936)," *Quipu: Revista Latinoamericana de Historia de las Ciencias y la Tecnología* 2 (1985): 95–122; "El Instituto de Medicina Social: Primeros intentos de institucionalizar la eugenesia," *Asclepio: Revista de Historia de la Medicina y de la Ciencia*, xl, 1 (1988): 343–58; and "Eugenesia y control social," *Asclepio*, xl, 2 (1988): 29–69. See also Mary Nash, "Ordenamiento jurídico y realidad social del aborto en España: Una aproximación histórica," in *Ordenamiento jurídico y realidad social de las mujeres: Siglos XVI a XX* (Madrid: Seminario de Estudios de la Mujer, Universidad Autónoma de Madrid, 1986), pp. 223–39. One of the few accounts of Italian eugenics I have come across is Claudio Pogliano, "Scienza e stirpe: Eugenica in Italia (1912–1939)," *Passato e Presente* 5 (1984): 61–97.

11. I have analyzed aspects of the Latin American medical tradition in several publications: *Beginnings of Brazilian Science: Oswaldo Cruz, Medical Research and Policy, 1890–1920* (New York: Science History Publications, 1976); "Initiation and Survival of Biomedical Research in a Developing Country: The Oswaldo Cruz Institute of Brazil, 1900–1920," *Journal of the History of Medicine and Allied Sciences* 30 (1975): 303–25; and "The Interplay between Socio-Economic Factors and Medical Science: Yellow Fever Research, Cuba, and the United States," *Social Studies of Science* 8 (1978): 397–423.

Latin American eugenics is of further comparative interest because Latin Americans were, to most eugenists situated outside the region, regarded as "tropical," "backward," and racially "degenerate." Not eugenic, in short. And yet Latin Americans had their own eugenic movements and activities. How then was eugenics defined? Who took it up and why? What social meanings got embedded in the science of heredity between the two world wars? What did "race" mean in a movement for racial improvement? All these questions are tied to the larger issue of how a sector of the intelligentsia in Latin America used the supposedly universal discourse of science to interpret modernity and progress.

I originally began my investigation with eugenics in Brazil. I found that there was much about eugenics, in its science and in its social style, that seemed unusual. First, the eugenists based their eugenics not on Mendelian conceptions of genetics, the dominant framework in Britain, the United States, and Germany, but on an alternative stream of Lamarckian hereditary notions. This style of eugenics reflected long-standing scientific connections with France as well as more local factors of political culture; it also helped structure debates about degeneration and determined how the new genetics and the sanitation sciences would interact in novel fashion in "eugenics." If Brazilian eugenics was distinctive in its scientific base, it was also distinctive in its application to the critical areas of reproduction and sexuality. In this first study I also began to explore how racial ideology in Brazil affected the way eugenics entered scientific discourse and social debate, and how eugenics became a source of interpretetive contention between various groups seeking to use eugenics for their different political projects. Since that first exploration of eugenics in Latin America, I have widened my net to include eugenics in several other parts of the region.[12]

In the last decades of the nineteenth century, eugenics emerged as an idea in many areas of Latin America as part of the debates about evolution, degeneration, progress, and civilization. But its more systematic development came after World War I, with the establishment of specific eugenics societies and organizations. Thereafter, eu-

12. Nancy Leys Stepan, "Eugenesia, genética y salud pública: El movimiento eugenésico brasileño y mundial," *Quipu: Revista Latinoamericana de Historia de las Ciencias y la Tecnología* 2 (1985): 351–84; and "Eugenics in Brazil, 1917–1940," in *Wellborn Science* [note 10], pp. 110–52.

genics touched or influenced the history of medicine, the family, maternity, population, criminology, public health, and social welfare. Many legislative efforts concerning human reproduction, the control of disease, and the regulation of immigration in Latin America can be fully understood only by taking into account eugenic concepts, which at the very least gave them their rhetorical structure and their medical-moral rationale. Eugenics was significant because it occupied the cultural space in which social interpretation took place, and because it articulated new and compelling images of health as a matter of heredity and race.

To enter the world of Latin American eugenics is to enter an unexplored area of human activity and political pressure and to discover forgotten languages of science. Strange fields of knowledge, with such curious and now discarded names as "puericulture," "maternology," "euphrenics," and "nipology," are brought back into view and a semiological terrain is reconstructed and surveyed.[13] Eugenics was a discursive project that provided a framework for cultural prescription and medical-moral investigation. It is this project that my book seeks to elucidate.

Science, Race, and Gender

Before outlining the plan of the book, however, I need to introduce some major concepts and related theoretical orientations that inform my empirical research. The concepts concern science, race, and gender, and my orientation to them is, broadly speaking, "constructivist." By drawing attention to these concepts and approaches, I believe we can rethink the meaning of eugenics as a social-medical movement of modern times.

First, I assume, along with many historians of science today, that science is a highly social activity and is not sealed off from the values of the society in which it is practiced. From the more traditional concern with the reconstruction of the internal coherence of major

13. Two contemporary accounts in French were M. T. Nisot, *La question eugénique dans divers pays* (Brussels: Librairie Faile, 1927), and Henri-Jean Marchaud, *L'évolution de l'idée eugénique* (Bordeaux: Imprimerie-Librairie de l'Université, 1933). A somewhat rare secondary (and late) account in Spanish by a Latin American is Roberto Mac-Lean y Estenos, *La eugenesia en América* (Mexico City: Instituto de Investigaciones Sociales, Cuadernos de Sociología, Imprenta Universitaria, 1952).

theories in science, historians have shifted their attention toward more sociological and/or naturalistic views of science as a product of culture and social life. Although interest in science as an internally consistent and internally driven kind of empirical knowledge has not disappeared, many historians have begun to explore science contextually and to examine the way elements of society conventionally considered external and only indirectly connected to science become constituent parts of scientific theories themselves, as well as of their associated scientific practices.[14] As a result, science reveals itself as much more contingent and culturally specific than it has been thought to be. This issue raises complex interpretive issues that cannot be gone into in detail here, but its application to an area of the human sciences like eugenics is clear.[15] Since eugenics was both a science and a social movement, it lends itself to a constructivist approach in which political and other factors surrounding the development and endorsement of particular genetic theories, and the social policies derived from them, can be explored. The study of eugenics allows historians to move from abstract notions about the possible social generation of scientific knowledge to more historically nuanced, locally specific studies of science in culture. This is the way I have examined eugenics in Latin America—first, as a science of heredity that was shaped by political, institutional, and cultural factors particular to the historical moment and place in which it appeared; and, second, as a social movement with an explicit set of policy proposals that appeared to their proponents to be suggested by, or be logically derived from, hereditarian science itself.

14. A convenient way of dating the "new" history of science is from the appearance in 1962 of Thomas S. Kuhn's book *The Structure of Scientific Revolutions* (Chicago: University of Chicago Press, 2d ed. 1972). Although Kuhn's work was primarily intellectualist in emphasis rather than sociological, it did raise new questions about the sociology of knowledge. For a review of the new sociology of science, with bibliography, see Michael Mulkay, "Sociology of Science in the West," *Current Sociology* 28(3) (1981): 1–184; for an account of the new social history of science see Steven Shapin, "History of Science and Its Sociological Reconstructions," *History of Science* 20 (1982): 157–211; realist, constructivist, and contextualist approaches to scientific knowledge are reviewed and analyzed by Karin D. Knorr-Cetina in her book *The Manufacture of Knowledge: An Essay on the Constructivist and Contextual Nature of Science* (London: Pergamon Press, 1981).

15. Some of the most interesting work in the sociology and social history of scientific theory, however, has been done in the physical sciences; an example is Andrew Pickering, *Constructing Quarks: A Sociological History of Particle Physics* (Chicago: University of Chicago Press, 1984).

A corollary of the new constructivist history of science is that historians no longer conceptualize science as depicting "reality" in any straightforward or transparent fashion but rather as constructing or creating the objects it studies and giving them their empirical weight and meaning. Genetics and eugenics, for example, created and gave scientific and social meaning to new objects of study, such as the supposed hereditarily unfit or "dysgenic" individuals or groups that constituted particular human populations. In this sense, science is seen as a productive force, generating knowledge and practices that shape the world in which we live. In this book, I explore how, through the science and social movement associated with the new field of genetics (a word coined in 1905), cultural meaning was encoded within and by science. Science carries immense social authority in the modern world—an authority based on its claim to facticity, neutrality, and universality. I hope to show how eugenics, perceived as a science, produced perceptions and techniques that shaped cultural interpretations and led to the development of social strategies.

Closely connected to these issues of scientific interpretation is the issue of race. As a science of "race improvement," some concept of race was of course built into eugenics from the start. At times "race improvement" meant merely the genetic improvement of "the human race" or "our people"; more often, however, eugenists were concerned with particular portions of the human population, which they perceived as being divided into distinct and unequal "races." Although no other eugenics movements went so far as the Nazis in exterminating races in the name of eugenics, most employed racist discourse as defined by Pierre-André Taguieff. Groups self-identified as dominant marked off other groups as inferior, through a language that asserted differences and created boundaries. These differences were presupposed to be fixed and natural (e.g., biological) and to limit each individual member to a fundamental "type." As a movement derived from ideas about biological heredity, eugenics provided a new set of conceptions and political principles with which to express and constitute differences within the social body.[16]

16. See Pierre-André Taguieff, "Racisme et antiracisme: Modèles et paradoxes," in *Racismes, antiracismes,* ed. André Béjin and Julien Freund (Paris: Librairie des Méridiens, 1986), pp. 253–302, and his book *La force du préjugé: Essai sur le racisme et ses doubles* (Paris: Editions la Découverte, 1988), esp. chaps. 8 and 9.

Eugenics was connected to another set of differences, those of sex and gender. Histories often mention that eugenics was related to women, but usually more in passing than as a central theme. This omission is surprising, since the novelty of eugenics as a scientific-social movement lay in its concentrated focus on human reproduction as the arena for the play of science and social policies. It aimed to identify the supposedly "dysgenic" features of the body or behavior caused by heredity in individuals and groups and to find social means to prevent bad heredity from continuing. Eugenists were especially concerned with women because they took reproduction to define women's social role far more than it did that of men; women were also more socially vulnerable and dependent than men, making management of their reproductive-hereditary lives seem more urgent and more possible. Eugenic prescriptions and proscriptions therefore fell differentially on men and women. In this book, I examine how eugenics defined biological and cultural distinctions of gender and how race and gender intertwined to construct new images and social practices of the "fit" nation.

In keeping with the social constructivist approach outlined earlier, I assume that racial and gender definitions are not "given" by nature but are historically constituted in different ways in different historical periods. In the case of gender, this assumption is based on the insight developed over the last several years by many scholars, notably feminist ones, that many of the things we think of as natural, "essential," or timeless facts of sexual difference are not the results of anatomy and physiology understood unproblematically and objectively by the inquiring mind of the neutral observer, but instead complicated and essentially social constructions connected to larger practices and institutions in society. Feminist scholars have introduced the word "gender" in English-language discussions precisely to indicate that our understanding of sexual differences, or the social and political roles taken to be appropriate to those differences, are not, as they have often been taken to be, obvious or based in simple ways on well-known differences of sexual physiology and anatomy. Sexual differences in reproduction are not enough to explain why women in the past have been denied the vote, excluded from certain kinds of work, and treated as legal minors. These aspects of women's lives are instead related to gender and are essentially political and normative, not biological and anatomical. Some feminists would go further to argue that even the seemingly most obvious facts of biology differentiating the sexes (e.g., hormone differences) are also socially constituted, so that gender assumptions are always part of our understanding of biological sex and vice versa.[17] I have used gender in this book to indicate that sexual differences are constructed most powerfully around naturalized social categories and that in this process of naturalization science has played a crucially important role.

No equivalent word to "gender" exists to indicate the socially constituted character of the "races" represented in European science and politics. Yet the argument for their politically and historically constructed character is compelling. Scientists' many disputes over racial classifications, and the inability to find a classification that would satisfy once and for all the requirement for authoritative ways to divide the human species into fixed types, are powerful indicators that racial categories are not representations of preexisting biological groups transparently understood but distinctions based on complex political-scientific and other kinds of conventions and discriminatory practices. Racial distinctions are not timeless but have constantly been renegotiated and experienced in different ways in different historical periods. We should think, then, of the races that constituted the objects of the movement of race improvement as "artifactual" aspects of the human sciences. I take this term to refer to an object of knowledge that is constructed as a biological and social "fact" grounded in what is taken to be empirical nature. At the same time, the term indicates that we do not experience human variation or human difference "as it really is, out there in nature," but by and through a system of representations which in essence creates the objects of difference. This book asks what part eugenics played in the construction of race and gender differences, and how gender and

17. These insights are the work of many authors. For a succinct summary of the feminist understanding of gender, see Joan Wallach Scott, *Gender and the Politics of History* (New York: Columbia University Press, 1988), esp. chap. 2. For a telling critique of the biological "facts" of sex difference, see especially Evelyn Fox Keller, "Women Scientists and Feminist Critics of Science," *Daedalus* 4 (Fall 1987): 77–92, and her "The Gender/Science System; or, Is Sex to Gender as Nature Is to Science?" *Hypatia* 2 (Fall 1987): 37–49. Along rather different lines, there is Anne Fausto-Sterling, *Myths of Gender: Biological Theories about Women and Men* (New York: Basic Books, 1985). See also Nelly Oudshoon, "On Measuring Sex Hormones: The Role of Biological Assays in Sexualizing Chemical Substances," *Bulletin of the History of Medicine* 64 (1990): 243–61, and my own article "Race and Gender: The Role of Analogy in Science," *Isis* 77 (1986): 261–77.

race discursively intertwined in the debates about identity and fitness.[18]

The Scope and Plan of the Book

I have made two choices about the scope of this book. First, I have viewed eugenics primarily through the prism of the movement itself. This book is a history, therefore, of the individuals, publications, and institutions of eugenics, in their prescriptive and proscriptive aspects. This choice was dictated by practical considerations, especially the novelty of my topic in Latin American studies and the lack of secondary materials on even closely related themes. By and large, histories of Latin American intellectual life and institutions, the professions, public health, and women—all matters having a bearing on my theme—are tasks for the next generation of scholars. I am especially sorry to have to leave for another book, or another historian, the study of the reactions of the people, most of them poor and many of them illiterate, who were the targets of the eugenists' ill-considered plans and policies. But by concentrating on the individuals and groups who self-consciously promoted scientific eugenics, I have been able to emphasize the political significance of the knowledge-claims of the eugenists in the areas of human heredity and health. I have been able, that is, to keep at the center of my analysis the problem of eugenics as a movement based on science or claiming legitimacy because of its connections to science. Throughout the book, in fact, issues relating to science and social action are kept in the foreground, to a degree perhaps not common in other historical studies of eugenics.

My second choice has been to focus on three Latin American countries as exemplary of eugenics in the region. The three are Bra-

---

18. The historical literature on race and race difference is large. An excellent starting point is Stephen Jay Gould's book *The Mismeasure of Man* (New York: Norton, 1981), where he explores the variety of ways "race" was created through scientific theory and practice in the nineteenth and early twentieth centuries. I also discuss races as historical-social constructions within science in *The Idea of Race in Science: Great Britain, 1800–1960* (London: Macmillan, 1982). In the introduction to that book, I discuss how "lowland Scots," "Celts," and "Mediterraneans" (to take only a few examples) were counted as biological races at various times in the nineteenth century. See also the analysis in my article "Biological Degeneration: Races and Proper Places," in *Degeneration: The Dark Side of Progress*, ed. J. Edward Chamberlin and Sander L. Gilman (New York: Columbia University Press, 1985), pp. 97–120. I first heard the term "artifactual" from Donna Haraway.

zil, Argentina, and Mexico. This selection has allowed me to explore enough Latin American examples to see whether a Latin family likeness in eugenics existed and to sort out some of the factors that might be connected to such a family. The analysis, then, is explicitly and implicitly comparative—explicitly within Latin America itself, and implicitly with Europe and the United States. The three countries chosen were the most populous in Latin America. Each had an organized interest in eugenics and all were sufficiently involved in the world of science to be selective users of hereditarian ideas and to adapt them to local interests and necessities.[19] At the same time, these countries differed sufficiently—in social structure, racial makeup and ideology, economic development and politics—to provide interesting comparisons within the Latin American setting.

Brazil was a leader in Latin America in the biomedical and sanitation sciences in the first two decades of the twentieth century, and the first to establish formally a eugenics society. Brazil's population was racially mixed, illiterate, and poor, and the country's small, largely European, intelligentsia had long been preoccupied with the racial identity and health of the nation when eugenics appeared on the scene. The notion that racial improvement could be achieved scientifically therefore had considerable appeal to medical doctors and social reformers. In these circumstances, the potential existed for an extreme race-hygiene movement; but so did political space for less extreme definitions of the meaning of eugenics for the nation.

Argentina, with Brazil, was the most advanced scientifically of the Latin American countries. It was also by far the wealthiest in the 1920s and 1930s. Racially, however, Argentina took its identity to be white, not mulatto or black; the Indian population of the country had been drastically reduced by violent campaigns of conquest and control; large-scale European immigration, mainly from Italy and Spain, had led to the idea that Argentina was a potential Europe in the Americas. In the circumstances, eugenic debate revolved mainly around which of the European "races" and which social classes best represented Argentine nationality and what could be done to make

19. The three are historically and currently the largest contributors to science from Latin America. See Patricia McLauchlan de Arregui, *Indiciadores comparativos de los resultados de la investigación científica y tecnológica en América Latina* (Lima, Peru: GRADE, 1988).

that nationality fit. Given the strong personal and institutional connections between Argentina and Mussolini's Italy in the 1930s, Argentina provides an important example of the ties between fascism and eugenics in Latin America.

Mexico stands out as the only country in Latin America to have undergone a profound social and political upheaval in the early twentieth century. The Mexican Revolution that began in 1910 shattered the old political arrangements, altered the ideological landscape, and transformed the national state. The revolutionary and secular setting of eugenics in Mexico was therefore very different from the setting in Brazil and Argentina. Yet if eugenics was associated with radicalism (and so revealed as not a monopoly of the right), Mexicans shared with other Latin Americans a deep concern with the health and racial makeup of their country. The country's semiofficial, revolutionary view of its population as biologically united in a superior, mestizo or "cosmic" race, in which merged all the different racial elements of the country, was undercut by the real political and social marginalization of the unacculturated Indians. Again a question is raised about what form eugenics would take in such circumstances.

The histories of eugenics in these three countries are organized thematically. Chapter 1 briefly introduces the scientific and political meaning of eugenics as it has normally been understood in Europe and North America and prepares the way for a different interpretation of eugenics in Latin America. In Chapter 2, I turn to Latin America as a setting for eugenics in the 1920s. With Brazil as my starting point, I analyze the political, social, and other factors that set the stage for eugenics ideologies and policies after World War I. I identify which individuals and groups embraced eugenics, where they were located professionally and socially, what kinds of institutions they established.

In Chapter 3, I explore in some detail how eugenics was first interpreted in the 1920s as a new kind of social hygiene. All three countries I examine were "postcolonial" and politically independent, yet they were bound up in the networks of the informal empires of Europe and the United States.[20] Long-standing cultural ties to France

20. The use of eugenics in colonial settings in the 1920s and 1930s is just beginning to be studied. A particularly interesting analysis is by Ann Laura Stoler, "Making the Empire Respectable: Race and Sexual Morality in Twentieth-Century Colonial Cultures," *American Ethnologist* 16 (1989): 634–60.

were especially important in suggesting a "soft" style of eugenics which was distinct from the "hard" Mendelian eugenics familiar to us from Britain and the United States. Genetics was not, in the period between 1900 and 1940, a monolithic or homogeneous body of knowledge; different approaches competed for scientific attention and political appropriation. Early on, eugenics in Latin America was associated theoretically with flexible neo-Lamarckian notions of heredity (in which no sharp boundaries between nature and nurture were drawn) and practically with public-health interventionism.

The outcome was a "preventive" eugenics directed to improving the nation by cleansing from the milieu those factors considered to be damaging to people's hereditary health. As a style, preventive eugenics extended the tradition of medical environmentalism into the new era of genetics and thereby did much to give eugenics its initial appeal to medical experts. Nonetheless, preventive eugenics did less to improve public health in Latin America (most of the eugenists' social-welfare recommendations were never implemented) than to promote new, biologically governed norms of social behavior which were justified in the name of hereditarian science—something new, modern, and in keeping with the scientific standards of Europe.

In Chapter 4, I turn to eugenics in the area of human reproduction. I explore what I call, borrowing from the Latin Americans themselves, "matrimonial eugenics." The germ plasm the eugenists believed to be altered for the worse by acquired heredity was transmitted to future generations in sexual reproduction. Some kind of control over the quality of that reproduction therefore became the goal of most eugenics movements. Here I am interested not just in the kinds of proposals the eugenists made but in the ways these proposals constructed gender, both female and male, in new terms. The issue of policies is additionally important because many of the radical and negative techniques suggested or legislated in eugenics in European countries and in the United States, notably human sterilization, were for religious and other reasons not publicly acceptable in the region. With some very significant and historically telling exceptions, they did not come to define the movement. At the same time, Latin American doctors and scientists wanted to develop new procedures, based on their understanding of heredity and health, for ensuring the hygiene of the reproductive cells of heredity and for creating fertile and fit populations to fill the empty spaces of their countries. Eugenics was a normalizing program concerned with rationalizing and purifying sexuality; how this program worked to shape the reproductive roles of men and women in the nation is the theme that concerns me here.

In Chapter 5, I examine the part eugenics played in Brazil, Argentina, and Mexico in structuring notions of inclusion and exclusion of various populations in the national body and in giving that body its ethnic identity. Gender helped articulate the notion of race and vice versa, since through reproduction the "racial types" supposedly making up the body politic were created. Although Europeans tended to lump the Latin American countries together as generally dysgenic and disagreeable places of biocultural degeneration, the countries actually varied considerably in the articulation of their racial ideologies and therefore in the racial inflections of their eugenics movements. Yet the movements were also united by a common concern, how to create out of their heterogeneous populations a new and purified homogeneity on which a true "nationhood" could be erected. Eugenics in Latin America developed coincidentally with the resurgence of various nationalisms, first in the aftermath of World War I, and again in the 1930s, in the wake of the worldwide depression and the ensuing severe dislocations and political mutations. In a time of worries about the racial foundations of their national identities, about the dangers to or possibilities for a perfected nationality provided by new immigrants, and about the negative effects caused by migrations of "inferior" types from the countryside into the cities, eugenists in Latin America found a role for scientific prescriptions and policy making.[21]

In Chapter 6, I consider Latin American eugenics in its international dimensions and connections. More specifically, I ask how eugenics became part of the political relations between nations, especially in debates about national identity and the flow of peoples across boundaries. I look closely at the Pan American experiment in eugenics, which brought eugenists from the United States into con-

21. Like many others, I have found Benedict Anderson's discussion of nationalism in his *Imagined Communities: Reflections on the Origin and Spread of Nationalism* (London: Verso, 1986) useful for my work. Anderson conceptualizes the nation as a relatively recent cultural artifact, which he associates with the appearance of modern nationalisms. Interestingly, however, Anderson denies that racism is connected to dreams of nationality (see chap. 8). I obviously disagree with him on this point. Jean Franco has also incorporated Anderson's ideas into her analysis of gender and women's writing in Mexico; see her *Plotting Women: Gender and Representation in Mexico* (New York: Columbia University Press, 1989).

tact with their Latin American counterparts and was intended to ensure Pan American cooperation in the field. The story of Pan American eugenics is a story of failure; rather than creating a powerful Code of Eugenics for the region, as some eugenists had hoped, only watered-down, compromise resolutions emerged from the two Pan American eugenics conferences held in the 1920s and 1930s. The story of this venture is interesting, however, because it made clear some of the differences separating U.S. and Latin American eugenists—in the definition of eugenics, its proper scope, and its political valuations. The story allows us to identify some of the special characteristics of the "family" of eugenics to which the Latin Americans believed they belonged. It also helps explain why the Latin International Federation of Eugenics Societies, founded in the 1930s, seemed to promise an attractive venue for Latin Americans because it was at once somewhat international—in that it established connections to Italy, France, and other European countries with whom the Latin Americans believed they shared a supposedly Latin culture—and yet not wholly international—in that it excluded the eugenics of "Anglo-Saxon" nations, which many Latin Americans opposed. The debate between supposed Anglo-Saxon practicality, materiality, and extremity and Latin humanity and sensibility was hardly new in Latin American history; but the story of Latin Americans' efforts to both participate in a modern scientific movement and resist particulars of its ideology unfavorable to themselves adds an interesting twist to the debate and to our understanding of eugenics. The fate of the Latin Federation—and indeed, the fate of eugenics generally in the late 1930s and 1940s as a movement with significant scientific and social weight—provides the coda to this chapter.

Chapter 7 reflects generally on eugenics as a powerful movement of biopolitics between the two world wars. I do not attempt to sort out the complicated history of human genetics after the war, when the field tried to reconstitute itself in a form uncontaminated by past eugenic ideas; this history is only now being taken up, and Latin American contributions to it are in any case marginal.[22] Nor do I try to compare the eugenics of the pre-1945 period with the social and ethical choices that face us today in the field of modern genetics.

22. The most detailed account of developments in human genetics after World War II, and of the emergence of the "new eugenics," is Kevles's in his *In the Name of Eugenics* [note 2], esp. chap. 17.

Rather, I pull together some of the conclusions that emerge from the history of eugenics in Latin America and use them as a springboard for some reflections on the relations between science and politics in different social and political settings. In particular, I examine the lessons of eugenics for what I call a "politics of scientific interpretation," a major theme of my book.

I

The New Genetics and
the Beginnings of Eugenics

Eugenics was hardly a new idea in 1883, despite the new name coined for it that year. In some ways the weeding out of unfit individuals went back to the Greeks, as British eugenists were fond of pointing out, perhaps because the association gave classical authority to the otherwise shocking notion that since not all individuals are equally endowed in nature not all should necessarily be allowed to reproduce themselves.

Nevertheless, "our" eugenics, properly speaking, belongs to the late nineteenth century and to the era of modern hereditarian science. The eventual enthusiasm for eugenics expressed by scientists, physicians, legal experts, and mental hygienists must be seen as the culmination of a long process of intellectual and social transformation in the nineteenth century, in which human life was increasingly interpreted as being the result of natural biological laws. Early in the century, for instance, Thomas Malthus, whose works on the "laws" of the biological inevitability of human overpopulation haunted nineteenth-century political economy, remarked that it did not by any means seem impossible that by selective breeding "a certain degree of improvement, similar to that amongst animals, might take place among men." He added, however, "As the human race could not be improved in this way, without condemning all the bad specimens to celibacy, it is not probable that an attention to breed should ever become general."[1]

The moral objections to the deliberate control of human breeding to improve the species seemed unanswerable, especially in the light of the inadequacy of knowledge of the matter or of the pattern of hereditary transmission. But as hereditarian explanations of both pathological and normal traits in human beings gained in popularity in mid-century, so protoeugenic speculations and proposals increased. For example, in 1850 the French scientist Prosper Lucas, in one of the most widely read studies of heredity of the period, drew up genealogical tables of the mental and moral characteristics of condemned criminals and urged the French government to discourage the perpetuation of such lineages, on the understanding that criminality would thereby be checked and French society improved permanently.[2] This example serves to remind us that negative eugenics did not depend on a specific theory of heredity, such as Mendelism, even though eugenic ideas became more acceptable as the consensus grew that the laws of heredity were actually understood.

New Theories of Heredity and Evolution

The new evolutionism of the 1860s was of great importance to the rise of eugenics in giving it a new scientific rationale and its indispensible terminology. The first assays into the dangerous territory of human hereditary and social policy by the "father" of eugenics himself, the scientist, traveler, geographer, and statistician Francis Galton, occurred in 1865 shortly after his reading of *The Origin of Species*. Evolution gave Galton ideas that, clustered together in a new fashion, formed the kernel of eugenics: the significance of hereditary variation in domestic breeding, the survival of the fittest in the struggle for life, and the analogy between domestic breeding and natural selection. The implications of natural and domestic selection for human society were worked out in more substantial, if substantially flawed, fashion in 1869 in *Hereditary Genius*, a book that still stands as the founding text of eugenics.

1. As quoted in J. Dupaquier et al., *Malthus Past and Present* (London: Academic Press, 1983), p. 268.
2. Example given by Frederick B. Churchill, in "Hereditary Theory to *Vererbung*: The Transmission Problem, 1850–1915," *Isis* 78 (1987): 342.

In this book, Galton took it upon himself to prove by simple genealogical and statistical methods that human ability was a function of heredity and not of education. From the demonstration of the part played by heredity in human talent, it seemed a relatively easy move from this knowledge to its social possibilities: "I propose to show in this book," said Galton in the very first sentence of his introduction, "that a man's natural abilities are derived by inheritance. . . . Consequently, as it is easy . . . to obtain by careful selection a permanent breed of dogs or horses, gifted with the peculiar powers of running, or of doing anything else, so it would be quite practicable to produce a highly gifted race of men by judicious marriages during several consecutive generations."[3]

Nevertheless, the path from hereditarianism in biosocial thought to the deliberate manipulation of the hereditary fitness of human populations was far from straight and narrow. Until the end of the nineteenth century moral and political distaste for interfering in human reproduction continued to prevent the translation of eugenic arguments into action. Galton's deductions from evolutionary biology intrigued but troubled Charles Darwin, for instance; Darwin cited Galton several times in his *Descent of Man*, but though he seemed at times to be on the brink of accepting the necessity for some kind of eugenic control over human reproduction in the name of evolutionary advancement, Darwin was reluctant about so radical a notion.[4] For most of his contemporaries, moral caution overrode the apparent logic of Galton's argument that, as civilization improved so that the weak and unfit were cared for, thereby diminishing the power of natural selection to eliminate the unfit, society should contemplate a deliberate *social* selection to protect future generations from biological unfitness.

By the end of the nineteenth century, however, attitudes began to change. The reasons for this were as much social as scientific. The last three decades of the nineteenth century saw growing economic competition among nations and the rise of new demands from previously marginalized groups. Working-class and feminist politics challenged the status quo. Socially, the optimism of the

3. Francis Galton, *Hereditary Genius* (1869; London: Julyan Friedmann, 1979), p. 1.
4. Charles Darwin, *The Descent of Man and Selection in Relation to Sex*, 2 vols. (London: John Murray, 1871), vol. 1, esp. pp. 167–84.

mid-Victorian period began to give way to widespread pessimism about modern life and its ills. Anxiety about the future progress of society was reinforced by unease about modernity itself. This anxiety provided the context in which a scientific movement of reform could develop. "Degeneration" replaced evolution as the major metaphor of the day, with vice, crime, immigration, women's work, and the urban environment variously blamed as its cause.[5] The belief that many of the diseases rife among the poor—tuberculosis, syphilis, alcoholism, mental illness—were hereditary merely fueled the fear of social decay. Many writers believed the "rapid multiplication of the unfit" to be a further threat.[6] Events seemed to be bearing out Galton's belief that the modern race was "over-weighted, and . . . likely to be drudged into degeneracy by demands that exceed its powers."[7] Meanwhile, the mysteries surrounding heredity seemed about to be solved by new conceptual and technical developments in science. From evolution, whose essence was the natural selection of inherited variations in animals and plants, Galton had concluded that society could do quickly what nature in the past had done more slowly, that is, improve the human stock by the deliberate selection of the fit over the unfit.[8] What was required to give such an idea weight in scientific circles was concrete knowledge of how heredity worked, a knowledge that was lacking when Galton first approached the subject of eugenics.

Then, in the 1890s, the German biologist August Weismann put forward his theory of the continuity of the "germ plasm," which indicated that there were theoretical and experimental grounds for thinking that only a portion of each cell carried hereditary material; moreover, Weismann proposed that the germ plasm was completely independent of the rest of the cell (the somaplasm) and that the germ plasm was inherited continuously by one generation from another without alteration from outside influences. Weismann's ideas challenged the long-standing notion of the inheritance of acquired characters associated with the French biologist Lamarck and his theory

5. For an analysis of the growth of the idea of degeneration, see *Degeneration: The Dark Side of Progress*, ed. J. Edward Chamberlin and Sander L. Gilman (New York: Columbia University Press, 1985).

6. This was the title of a book written by Victoria Woodhull in 1891.

7. Galton, as quoted in Dupaquier, *Malthus Past and Present* [note 1], p. 345.

8. R. J. Halliday calls the eugenists true Darwinians "in assimilating the biological problem of survival to the social problem of reproduction." See his "Social Darwinism: A Definition," *Victorian Studies* 14 (1971): 389–405.

of transmutation. In the Lamarckian tradition it was assumed that external influences on an individual life could permanently alter the germ plasm, so that the distinction between germ plasm and soma-plasm was blurred. As a theory of inheritance, the inheritance of acquired characters had long been commonplace in biology—it was in fact the standard explanation of how heredity worked.[9]

Galton had been convinced since the 1860s that Lamarckian ideas were wrong, in part because of his socially based conviction that the "genius" or intellectual success enjoyed by people like himself was unconnected to the educational and other social opportunities he enjoyed. He preferred to believe that social eminence was due to an inherited fitness that no amount of social engineering could affect and that was passed on from generation to generation by biological inheritance. His own genealogy, which linked him to the Darwins and the Wedgwoods, successful families of Victorian Britain, gave personal satisfaction and inner conviction of the correctness of his view that ability and success were primarily matters of biological history.

Several historians have analyzed the complicated social roots of Galton's eugenic argument; what is significant to our story is the way the language of "disinterested" science disguised those roots.[10] It is in fact only one of many examples in the history of the natural sciences in which issues that are social and political in character get "scientized" (to use an ugly neologism) so that they may claim an apolitical identity from which are later drawn highly political conclusions that have considerable authority precisely because they are based on apparently neutral knowledge.[11] The result was not a pseudoscience in any simple sense, since Galton stood squarely in a recognized scientific tradition and was a fully paid-up member, as it

9. On this point see Peter Bowler, *The Eclipse of Darwinism: Anti-Darwinian Evolution Theories in the Decades around 1900* (Baltimore: The Johns Hopkins University Press, 1983), chap. 4.

10. See especially Ruth Schwartz Cowan, "Nature and Nurture: The Interplay of Biology and Politics in the Work of Francis Galton," *Studies in the History of Biology* 1 (1977): 133–207; and Daniel Kevles, *In the Name of Eugenics: Genetics and the Uses of Human Heredity* (New York: Knopf, 1985), chap. 1.

11. The historical creation of our modern scientific epistemology of neutrality, objectivity, and universality, and the ideological functions of this epistemology are profoundly important topics in the history of science which are rarely explored. Aspects of the story in the case of Britain are analyzed in an excellent book by Jack Morrell and Arnold Thackray, *Gentlemen of Science: Early Years of the British Association for the Advancement of Science* (Oxford: Clarendon Press, 1981); see especially chap. 5.

were, of the scientific establishment. In many respects the way social values constructed a language of human variation and selection was typical, rather than otherwise, of the human social and biological sciences of the period.

What is also important to the history of eugenics is that Weismann's work, which was based on careful consideration of the problems of evolution and heredity, tended to confirm the movement toward the rejection of Lamarckian beliefs. Many biologists adopted his ideas with enthusiasm for this reason, thus strengthening the hereditarian strain in biological and social thought.

A few years after Weismann's work appeared, there followed the rediscovery in 1900 of Gregor Mendel's laws of the independent assortment and recombination of hereditary characters in plants. The stability of the Mendelian characters during genetic crosses and their reappearance in the next several generations unchanged, in definite numerical ratios, seemed to confirm Weismann's notion of the autonomy and inviolability of the germ plasm in which the hereditary material was carried. Mendelism offered the possibility that the simple numerical ratios discovered in plants would be found in animals and, by extension, in the human species.[12] Within a few years, the new science of "genetics" was defined and developed rapidly with the chromosome theory, the idea of the gene, and the use of statistical and biometric studies to become the foundation stone of modern genetics and evolutionary biology as we know them.[13] Mendelism thus represented a landmark in the development of modern biology.

Eugenics Movements in Europe and the United States

Eugenics as a social movement was shaped decisively by these developments. Even before 1900, scientists had begun to advance the idea that society should recognize the power of heredity in its social laws, in such a way as to favor reproduction of the physically and

12. Among the first demonstrations of Mendelian ratios in inheritance was Archibald Garrod's work on the recessive condition of alcaptonuria; see Alexander G. Bearn and Elizabeth D. Miller, "Archibald Garrod and the Development of the Concept of Inborn Errors of Metabolism," *Bulletin of the History of Medicine* 53 (Fall 1979): 315–27.

13. For these developments, see chapter 5 of my book *The Idea of Race in Science: Great Britain, 1800–1960* (London: Macmillan, 1982), pp. 111–39.

The New Genetics and Eugenics · 27

morally eugenical over the noneugenical.[14] Now that a science of
human heredity seemed at hand, moral objections to the social control of human reproduction received less weight. Nonetheless, the
correct social conclusions to be drawn from Weismann's theory of
heredity were not immediately obvious. Because science is never
unambiguous in its social messages, the meaning of this theory for
social policy was a matter of interpretation and was open to several
possibilities. If Weismann's ideas about the continuity of the germ
plasm were right, then the effects of education and improved surroundings would not be assimilated genetically over successive generations. Each new generation would have to start over, in hereditary terms, *de novo*. This result in turn could be read in two ways:
good genetic qualities could be found in all elements of the human
population, including the lower classes; or those found at the top of
the social pile were, in effect, the naturally best endowed genetically. Weismann could be read, that is, either optimistically or
pessimistically, radically or conservatively, positively or negatively.
All these kinds of readings are found in the literature of the period.

The fear in Europe and the United States about social degeneration, about the alterations brought about by industrialization, urbanization, migration, immigration, about changing sexual mores and
women's work, gradually led the more negative social interpretation
of Weismannism to predominate. Socially successful individuals and
groups were taken to be genetically and innately well endowed; the
poor and unsuccessful were viewed as products of poor heredity. In
most countries where Weismannism and Mendelism thrived, alternative interpretations were eventually marginalized in social-eugenic
debate. Henry Fairfield Osborn, the director of the American Museum of Natural History, spoke of the need to select "the fittest
chains of race plasma"; he was typical in moving in the 1890s from
an initially sanguine view of Weismannism to a pessimistic and conservative eugenic interpretation of human heredity.[15] When Mendel

14. Kevles, *In the Name of Eugenics* [note 10], chap. 4.
15. Henry Fairfield Osborn, "The Present Problem in Heredity," *Atlantic Monthly*
67 (March 1891): 354. Michael Freeden, in his book *The New Liberalism: An Ideology
of Social Reform* (Oxford: Clarendon Press, 1978), pp. 88–89, gives examples of progressive interpretations of Weismann's new theory, in which people emphasized that
good "nature" could be found at the bottom of the social scale as well as the top and
that with good environments and education such natures could have a chance to
develop fully.

was rediscovered in 1900, his ideas on inheritance were easily assimilated into the eugenic outlook. Since Mendelism, when combined with Weismann's theory of the autonomy of the germ plasm, was associated with the idea of the complete separation of hereditary units from environmental influences, to many scientists it seemed that no amount of tinkering with the social environment would result in long-lasting improvement of hereditary traits. Ancestry, rather than social life, was taken to determine character; heredity was now all. Indeed, simply calling a trait, condition, or behavior "hereditary" rather than "social" in origin seemed to imply a host of specific conclusions—that the condition was somehow "in" the individual in a way that something socially caused was not, that it was "fixed" in a peculiarly damaging manner, that there was nothing much that could be done about it short of trying to prevent the condition from being handed on through reproduction to future generations. Karl Pearson, the British scientist who became the first recipient of the new Galton eugenics professorship at University College, London University, put it with characteristic bluntness: "No degenerate and feebleminded stock will ever be converted into healthy and sound stock by the accumulated effects of education, good laws and sanitary surroundings. We have placed our money on environment when heredity wins by a canter."[16]

As confidence grew in many places that heredity was a fixed quantity at birth which determined a large range of human behaviors, eugenics societies began to be formed, some with the goal of pursuing scientific investigations of genetics in a scholarly and scientific fashion, others to discuss and promote new policies and even legislation in support of eugenic ideas. The first was the German Society for Race Hygiene, founded in Berlin in 1905; then came the Eugenics Education Society in England in 1907–1908, the Eugenics Record Office in the United States in 1910, and the French Eugenics Society in Paris in 1912. Outside specifically eugenics organizations, eugenic themes found their way into scientific areas such as anthropology, psychiatry, and sociology; eugenics sections were established in many of the organizations representing these disciplines.

Some biologists recognized the dangers of erecting social policies on incomplete knowledge.[17] Eugenics was on the whole a minority,

16. Quoted in B. Semmel, *Imperialism and Social Reform* (London: Allen and Unwin, 1960), p. 48.
17. See for instance the cautionary note sounded by the geneticist R. C. Punnett

professional and specialized point of view. Some of the legislation proposed by eugenists was radical enough to be actively resisted, especially in those countries where the public-health tradition was strong and public-health officials had a vested interest in defending their environmentalist approach against the new biological view of health.[18] On the other hand, the notion that the state had an interest in regulating the health and fitness of populations was well established in Europe and the United States, while Darwinian and agricultural approaches to improving stocks prepared the ground for extending the farming metaphors and practices to human populations.[19]

Eugenists were therefore not deterred from putting forward ideas about the control of human reproduction which would have struck such luminaries of biology as Thomas Henry Huxley and Alfred Russel Wallace as intolerable only a few decades before. Many eugenists believed the evidence that differences between individuals or groups depended on organic inheritance was sufficient to conclude that selective breeding was *the* key to human improvement. As the British eugenist Wicksteed Armstrong put it in his book *The Survival of the Unfittest* in 1930: "to diminish the dangerous fertility of the unfit there are three methods: the lethal chamber, segregation and sterilization."[20]

Actually, eugenists recommended a host of social policies as apparently logical deductions from hereditarian science, most of them not nearly as extreme as involuntary sterilization or euthanasia; their suggestions ranged from child and family allowances for the eugenically fit, to segregation of the unfit, to eugenic selection of im-

in 1912 in "Genetics and Eugenics," his paper at the first International Eugenics Congress; in *Problems in Eugenics* (London: Eugenics Education Society, 1912), p. 138.

18. Several historians have commented on the resistance of medical-health officers working in schools and similar institutions in Britain, where there was by the early twentieth century a strong public-health tradition; see especially G. R. Searle, "Eugenics and Class," in *Biology, Medicine, and Society, 1840–1940*, ed. C. Webster (Cambridge: Cambridge University Press, 1981), pp. 217–42; and Dorothy Porter, "'Enemies of the Race': Biologism, Environmentalisms, and Public Health in Edwardian England," *Victorian Studies* 34 (Winter 1991): 159–178.

19. The agricultural-eugenic connection was especially important in the United States; see Barbara A. Kimmelman, "The American Breeders' Association: Genetics and Eugenics in an Agricultural Context, 1903–1913," *Social Studies of Science* 13 (1983): 163–204.

20. Quoted in Margaret Canovan, *G. K. Chesterton: Radical Populist* (New York: Harcourt Brace Jovanovich, 1977), p. 66.

migrants. But by the late 1920s many eugenists had shifted their attention from the "positive" eugenics imagined by Galton, which favored incentives for the reproduction of the fit, to a "negative" eugenics that aimed to prevent reproduction of the unfit.[21] The lower classes breeding in the slums, the permanently unemployed, the poor alcoholics, the mentally ill sequestered in insane asylums—and their supposed hereditary unfitnesses—were now targets of eugenists' agitation. Daniel Kevles says, moreover, that by 1930 human sterilization had become for many eugenists the "paramount programmatic interest."[22] The introduction of the idea of compulsory sterilization of the unfit was also, of course, by far the most dramatic alteration in the traditional norms governing the Western family and individual rights to reproduction. Although regulation of sexuality and reproduction by the state already had a long history by the end of the nineteenth century (e.g., in the medical regulation of prostitution), this new proposal was a radical departure for public policy.

It is important to stress that the deliberate sterilization of human beings was put forward as a logical conclusion derived from genetics long before the Nazi eugenic program came into effect and that it was not always a proposal of the political right. The first eugenic sterilization laws in Europe were introduced in the canton of Vaud in Switzerland in 1928 and in Denmark in 1929 and were viewed as moderate, scientific, and progressive methods of implementing genetic hygiene. Although the Danish doctors rejected the racist idea of "Nordic" superiority which had become associated with much of German eugenics, according to the geneticist Tage Kemp the 1929 law was justified by the belief that "society must make living conditions tolerable for everybody, and this has necessitated the employment of certain eugenic measures."[23] According to a recent analysis, over eight and a half thousand Danes were sterilized for sexual and psychic abnormality between 1930 and 1949. In Sweden, where the

21. Galton had recommended competitive examinations to determine ability, encouragement of marriage within the selected group to ensure that offspring of the able reached full potential, and a system of grants for the fit. He advocated that the unfit be placed in monasteries and convents.

22. Kevles, *In the Name of Eugenics* [note 10], p. 393.

23. Tage Kemp, "Danish Experiments in Negative Eugenics, 1929–1945," *Eugenics Review* 38 (1945–1947): 182; see also Soren Hansen, "Eugenics Abroad II—In Denmark," *Eugenics Review* 23 (1931–1932): 234.

state-supported Institute for Race Biology was established in 1921 in connection with the University of Uppsala, at least fifteen thousand mental patients were eventually sterilized for eugenic reasons under the law passed in 1934 and put into effect the next year, the practice ending only after the war. Alva Myrdal, remembered as a pioneer of modern population policies, called in 1935 for a strengthening of the sterilization laws, which she regarded not as a method of preserving Swedish "racial quality" (since she believed that the fertility of the "social substratum" was not high) but as a means of protecting against individual suffering caused by bad heredity.[24] Technically, sterilization under the bill was voluntary; in practical terms, however, it was more or less involuntary.

But if any one country led the way in eugenic legislation before the 1930s it was the United States. The first U.S. state sterilization laws dated back to the first decade of the twentieth century. By the late 1920s, twenty-four states had passed involuntary sterilization laws, which were used to sterilize mainly the poor (and often black) inmates of institutions for the feeble-minded.[25] Even though the application of these laws was at times resisted and challenged, by the mid-1930s at least thirty thousand individuals had been sterilized under them; new sterilization laws were added in the late 1930s, and the number of sterilizations increased. Altogether, some seventy thousand individuals were sterilized in the United States between 1907 and the end of World War II.[26]

The most comprehensive sterilization law was of course that of Nazi Germany. Passed on July 14, 1933, following the dismissal from official posts of many of the Jewish and/or left-wing individuals who had been involved in eugenics and radical sexual reform issues in the Weimar Republic, the new legislation took eugenic sterilization in the Western world further by a whole order of magnitude (it had been forbidden in Germany until this date). The conditions labeled as hereditary and therefore covered by the terms of the 'Law for the Prevention of Genetically Diseased Offspring'

24. See Alva Myrdal, *Nation and Family* (London: Kegan Paul, Trench, Tubner, 1945), passim. Figures for the Danish sterilizations given by Stephen Trombley, *The Right to Reproduce: A History of Coercive Sterilization* (London: Weidenfeld and Nicolson, 1988), p. 159.
25. Kevles, *In the Name of Eugenics* [note 10], p. 111.
26. Ibid., p. 116; and Barry Mehler, "The New Eugenics," *Science for the People* 15 (May/June 1983): 18–23.

included "hereditary feeblemindedness," schizophrenia, manic depressive insanity, "hereditary epilepsy," Huntington's chorea, hereditary blindness and deafness, serious bodily deformity, and alcoholism. In his recent study of "racial hygiene" under the Nazis, Robert Proctor points out that all of these conditions were assumed either to be caused by single Mendelian characters or to be clear enough in their behavioral or physical manifestations to be treated by the law as though they were. Later, mixed-race offspring were added to the list of those to be sterilized. The law called for involuntary sterilization, and though appeal against sterilization was theoretically possible, very few appeals (3 percent) were actually granted. Proctor estimates that by 1945 the special genetic health courts established by the Nazis had ordered and supervised the involuntary sterilization of one percent of the entire German population.[27]

The Selective Appropriation of Science

This short survey encapsulates eugenics as generally understood—a scientific movement associated with social Darwinism and Mendelism, and a social program favoring the direct control of human reproduction over the more indirect methods of human improvement through reform of the environment. Although its proponents spanned the political spectrum from the left to the right, on the whole eugenics has been studied as a conservative movement of white, middle-class, Anglo-Saxon Protestants who believed themselves, and were seen by others, to be the most "fit" for procreation, individually and racially.

Given its espousal by well-known scientific and medical figures in Europe, eugenics appeared to have sound credentials, and the idea quickly made its way into the scientific reform agendas of many countries, including those in Latin America. The spread of science, from an originating point in Europe to areas beyond its boundaries, has long interested scholars concerned with the role of science and technology in creating empires or in stimulating industrial develop-

27. Robert N. Proctor, *Racial Hygiene: Medicine under the Nazis* (Cambridge: Harvard University Press, 1988), chap. 4.

ment in poor nations.[28] Underlying the notion of "spread," however, is an implicitly diffusionist model that rests on assumptions about "time lags" and "catching up" in science, as though the stages of science were already mapped out in advance by countries "further ahead" in the march of science. Diffusionism (or imperialism, another analytic framework that is more attentive to agency and power) tends to deflect attention from local sources of adaptation and the processes of selection involved when groups incorporate scientific theories and outlooks into their own traditions and institutions. As I remarked in the Introduction, ideas do not keep fixed identities as they travel through space and time; nor do they occupy previously empty social or intellectual spaces. They are rather complex parts of social life, generated within that social life, reflective of it, and capable of affecting it. Evolution meant different things in England than in France; Einstein's relativity acquired a different signification in Italy than in the United States. Ideas, even scientific ones, are always selectively reconfigured across cultural frontiers and the result is a science subtly shaped by local traditions—cultural, political, and scientific. We need, then, to study eugenics in places like Latin America not as a pale reflection of eugenics elsewhere, something perhaps "misunderstood" or "misinterpreted," but as something rooted in the region's own cultural experience and history.[29] Studied this way, Latin American eugenics can throw considerable light on the scientific foundations of social thought and the social construction of science.

"Defamiliarizing" eugenics in this way has the further advantage of highlighting for us a generic problem in the study of science and social life, namely, how scientific theories get connected to policy outcomes. Although a scientific theory may provide a social and cognitive basis for many social policies, the theory itself leaves many policy conclusions unspecified. The story of genetics in Latin America indicates that at any one time a scientific theory opens up several social possibilities while closing off others. Contestations about the proper meaning of a theory for social life are the norm, contesta-

28. George Basalla, in a pioneering article written many years ago, proposed a general model for understanding the diffusion of Western science: "The Spread of Western Science," *Science* 156 (1967): 611–22.

29. On these points, see especially Thomas F. Glick, "Cultural Issues in the Reception of Relativity," in *The Comparative Reception of Relativity*, ed. Thomas F. Glick (Leiden: D. Reidel, 1987), pp. 381–400.

tions whose outcomes cannot be decided a priori by reference to the science itself, as though it forced upon its users only some social conclusions and not others. Thus we will see that some eugenists who interpreted genetics in a soft, non-Mendelian fashion concluded that there was a place for traditional, environmental approaches to the reform of human heredity; others, equally sure that heredity worked by the inheritance of acquired characteristics, concluded that an environmentalist approach would be too slow to effect human improvement and that only radical controls over reproduction would bring about the desired results. Social conclusions are determined by a variety of contingent and local factors, such as the strategic location of different groups in political, intellectual and institutional life, their capacity to claim competency over a technical language (such as the language of genetics), or the perceived legitimacy of that language—that is, by social and political relations in society.

In short, social styles and social ideologies are not the predictable outcomes of the inherent logic of science. This is not at all to say that the science of heredity—or any theory of nature—is therefore ideologically neutral. It is to say, rather, that "nature," or the science that as a human practice produces it, does not escape the value conflicts existing in its social surroundings. As Ted Benton says in a different context, inferences from science are therefore not merely extrapolated but socially constructed.[30] It is useful to bear this in mind when we look at the meaning of heredity and eugenics in the various regions of the world.

30. My analysis follows Ted Benton's in "Social Darwinism and Socialist Darwinism in Germany: 1860 to 1900," *Revista di Filosofia* 73 (1982): 79–121. For other discussions of the range of social and political interpretations that could be associated with Darwinism, see James Allen Rogers, "Darwin and Social Darwinism," *Journal of the History of Ideas* 33 (1967): 389–405, and Nancy Leys Stepan, "Nature's Pruning Hook: War, Race, and Evolution, 1914–1918," in *The Political Culture of Modern Britain*, ed. John M. W. Bean (London: Hamish Hamilton, 1987), pp. 129–45.

2

Eugenics in Latin America: Its Origins and Institutional Ecology

This chapter maps out the social and political parameters of eugenics in Latin America. The metaphor of "ecology" employed in the chapter title draws attention to the fact that knowledge forms a complex and interrelated system that cannot be understood apart from its surrounding circumstances.[1] I emphasize the story in Brazil, perhaps the most complex of cases; I then bring in developments in Argentina and Mexico, and even on occasion in other countries in the region, in order to demonstrate that interest spanned the hemisphere and to identify some of the variations that occurred within eugenics according to local circumstances.

The Social, Scientific, and Ideological Context

Reference to eugenics in Latin American medical and social writings predate World War I.[2] But the Brazilian term "eugenía," as dis-

---

1. This ecology refers to the kinds of professional groups involved in eugenics, their scientific orientation, their relationships to political culture, and their connections to other groups and/or organizations concerned with the management of health. Italian eugenics, for example, was apparently much more closely connected to demography and sociology than was the case with eugenics in the United States. In Latin America, eugenics was medical and medico-legal in composition.

2. For example, eugenics was discussed in the 1880s in Argentina; see Chapter 3.

tinct from the Spanish American "eugenesia," was introduced as the title of a medical thesis in 1914.[3] The founding of the first Brazilian eugenics society in early 1918 (and one in Argentina a few months later), only ten years after the equivalent British society and six years after the French, suggests how attuned scientists in the region were to European developments. Structurally and socially, however, the origins of the eugenics movements related less to European than to Latin American factors.

One factor was World War I and its significance to Latin Americans. Brazil was the only country in Latin America actually to enter the war on the side of the allies, although many Latin American countries felt the economic and intellectual impact of the war. The European countries had long been symbols of all that was supposedly civilized and advanced, compared to Latin America's so-called barbarism and backwardness. The collapse of these European countries into their own barbarisms helped generate a new nationalism in many areas of Latin America, based on a desire to project the Latin American nation-states onto the world stage, to define the realities of the region concretely in Latin American terms instead of European ones, and to find Latin American solutions to Latin American problems. Whereas in Europe the war intensified fears about national degeneration, in Latin America the war created a new determination to bring about national regeneration. Throughout the 1920s, eugenics was associated with patriotism and the call for a larger role for Latin America in world affairs. In Brazil, more specifically, the subjects of wartime readiness and discipline, of control and order, of Brazilian capacities and racial capabilities, were much on the minds of the elites.[4]

3. Alexandre Tepedino, *Eugenía (esboço)* (Rio de Janeiro: Faculdade de Medicina, 1914). The term "eugenía" had been proposed by the Brazilian philologist João Ribeiro, in preference to the other word canvassed in Portuguese, "eugénica," which some scientists and grammarians suggested. See Renato Kehl, *Lições de eugenía* (Rio de Janeiro: Editor Brasil, 1935), p. 15. The term "eugenía" was further distinguished by the accent over the *i* (not usual in a word of this kind), perhaps to emphasize its similarity to the French word "eugénique," which also has its stress at the end. The word also appeared in a pamphlet, *Pro-eugenía*, by Magalhães in 1914. See M. T. Nisot, *La question eugénique dans les divers pays* (Brussels: Librairie Faile, 1927), pp. 207–13.

4. The impact of World War I on middle-class attitudes in Brazil, especially in relation to discipline and control, is discussed in *O Brasil republicano*, ed. Boris Fausto (São Paulo: Difel, 1978), vol. 3, pt. 2: 401–26.

Optimism, on the other hand, was necessarily tempered by the recognition that the problems facing Latin America were considerable indeed. A second factor influencing the development of eugenics was what we might call the crisis of "underdevelopment." The changes that had occurred in the region between 1870 and 1914 were massive. In Brazil, for example, socially the period encompassed the final collapse of a slave-based society in 1888 (the last such society in the Western world) and the opening up of the country to European immigration on a vast scale. Politically, the period saw the abolition of the monarchy and the creation of the republic in 1889. Economically, it witnessed Brazil's ever-deepening involvement in the world capitalist system, an involvement that kept Brazil in a position of dependence at the periphery, as a supplier of raw materials such as coffee. The consequences of such growth were often devastating—a skewed and "dependent" development whose social manifestations were poverty, social unrest, and often increasing rather than decreasing inequality, especially for the black and mulatto segments of the population. Brazil entered the twentieth century a highly stratified society, socially and racially—a society that, though formally a liberal republic, was governed informally by a small, largely white elite and in which less than 2 percent of the population voted in national elections; a society in which the majority of the people were black or mulatto and could not read or write; in which, though there was technical separation of church and state, Catholicism had considerable cultural influence; and in which democratic liberalism was seen by many intellectuals as irrelevant or harmful to Brazil's future.

By the second decade of the twentieth century, the appalling misery and ill health of the poor had crystallized in public consciousness as a national issue—as "the social question."[5] The group that most agitated physicians, sanitation experts, and reformers in Brazil was largely black and mulatto; these professionals assumed that social ills accumulated at the bottom of the racial-social hierarchy—that the poor were poor because they were unhygienic, dirty, ignorant, and hereditarily unfit. Racial and class biases thus merged in the language of heredity. In Brazil, the former slaves, the last 700,000 of

5. This was the title of Rui Barbosa's lecture in 1919, reprinted as *A questão social e política no Brasil* (Rio de Janeiro: Organização Simões, 1951). Many other books in Latin America from this period carried the same or similar titles.

whom had been emancipated as late as 1888, had been left without education or recompense, to compete on unfavorable terms for wage labor with the more than one and a half million white immigrants who entered the country between 1890 and 1920. One result of the wave of migration and immigration was the relatively sudden spurt of urbanism in Brazil. The population of the city of São Paulo, for instance, jumped from only 129,409 people in 1893 to 240,000 by 1900—a growth of nearly 100 percent in seven years. By 1907, Italians alone outnumbered Brazilians in the city by two to one. The federal capital to the northeast, Rio de Janeiro, was by this date a city nearing 800,000. Although both cities had undergone extensive remodeling and "civilizing"—grand boulevards created in the Parisian style, slums pushed to the outskirts, new middle-class areas established—and although both cities had improved the public sanitation services concerned with epidemic diseases, endemic diseases were left untreated, and general morbidity remained high.[6] The general standards of housing and sanitation of all but the still small middle class and elite sectors of the city remained extremely bad, and the state-led, often authoritarian programs of sanitation at times provoked resistance on the part of the poor.[7]

The perception and interpretation of social change were features of most eugenics movements. But in Brazil change was occurring in an extremely poor, socially and racially stratified, mainly rural, illiterate, and diseased country without any of the social-welfare legislation—the eight-hour working day, the prohibition of child labor, unemployment protection—that had become more or less standard in many parts of Europe by the early twentieth century.

Poverty, migration, immigration, and unemployment helped usher in a period of radicalized politics, protests, work stoppages, and strikes in the second decade of the twentieth century. In Brazil, this unrest climaxed in the first national strike in 1917, when forty thousand workers closed the city of São Paulo; medical doctors

6. The campaigns against epidemic disease are described in Nancy Stepan, *Beginnings of Brazilian Science: Oswaldo Cruz, Medical Research and Policy, 1890–1920* (New York: Science History Publications, 1981), chaps. 2 and 3.

7. See Jeffrey D. Needell, "The *Revolta Contra Vacina* of 1904," *Hispanic American Historical Review* 67 (May 1987): 233–69, and his book *A Tropical Belle Epoque: Elite Culture and Society in Turn-of-the-Century Rio de Janeiro* (Cambridge: Cambridge University Press, 1987), esp. chap. 1; and Teresa Meade, "'Living Worse and Costing More': Resistance and Riot in Rio de Janeiro, 1890–1917," *Journal of Latin American Studies* 21 (May 1989): 241–66.

made the first formal call for eugenics that same year, indicating how eugenics presented itself as a suprapolitical, medical path to ease the social tensions within a rapidly growing, urban population. The strike demonstrated the political potential of a newly emerging industrial working class, but it also demonstrated the weakness of organized labor and the power of the municipal and state authorities to use the police and militia to put down unrest ruthlessly, as British and North American visitors remarked. Traditionally, the educated, mainly white, elite feared violence and danger from blacks and mulattos, whom they portrayed as lazy, undisciplined, sickly, drunk, and in a constant state of vagabondage. To these fears were now added new ones about disorder and violence by foreign-born factory workers, many of whom were expelled from the country on charges of being anarchists bent on overthrowing the social order.[8]

The threat of urban unrest called into question the adequacy of old-style, laissez-faire liberalism for solving social problems and suggested new roles for the state in regulating relations between workers and owners and even in intervening directly in social life. In contrast to British eugenics, which constituted in part a response to the perception that years of social-welfare legislation had failed to improve the mental, physical, and moral conditions of the poor, Latin American eugenics was associated with the call for the introduction of such social legislation, and this association influenced the form it took.[9] Actual progress was pitifully slow in coming, and much of the social legislation eventually passed in the 1920s was more symbolic than real, an occasion for rhetoric rather than for any serious redistribution of economic and social resources.

A third factor in the rise of eugenics was the state of Latin American science. Eugenics in Latin America was not usually associated, as it was in Britain, with controversies concerning the relative merits of biometrics and Mendelian genetics. Even by the 1920s, Darwinian biology and the new genetics, as sources of biological research rather than cultural metaphors, involved only small groups of scientists. Brazil was untypical in Latin America in having no

8. Boris Fausto, "Controle social e criminalidade em São Paulo: Um apanhado geral (1890–1924)," in *Crime, violência e poder*, ed. Paulo Sergio Pinheiro (São Paulo: Brasiliense, 1983), pp. 193–210.

9. For the relationship between the supposed failures of social-welfare legislation and the development of British eugenics, see Nancy Stepan, *The Idea of Race in Science: Great Britain, 1800–1960* (London: Macmillan, 1982), pp. 117–18.

universities as such until the 1920s; the first modern university, properly speaking, was in fact not established until 1934. Biological work was therefore confined largely to the medical schools, agricultural institutes, and public-health organizations funded by federal and state agencies.

Nevertheless, if Latin Americans were still small contributers to science by world standards, the history of eugenics in the region must be seen as part of a generalized endorsement of science, as a sign of cultural modernity, and as a means by which the various countries of Latin America could emerge as powerful actors on the world scene. The period 1880 to 1930 was one of considerable intellectual growth and institutional consolidation in science. Just as the United States began to lose its cultural provincialism and develop institutions of modern science in the 1840s and 1850s, so in Latin America a few decades later science became a rallying cry for the modern, secular elite. In this period the scientific community acquired its national form and traditions. Scientists strove to develop technical skills and create societies that would encourage new, scientific outlooks; they worked to develop national surveys of their natural resources and contracted foreign specialists to aid them in undertaking programs of education and research. They established organizations with a practical rather than a literary bent which could help them expand agricultural production, deal with disease, clean up their cities, and exploit their natural riches. In Brazil, for instance, the Brazilian Society of Science was founded in Rio in 1916 to provide a new forum for the discussion and promotion of science.[10]

More generally, science was widely recognized as essential to Western material and cultural authority—to the very definition of modernity and civilization. Latin American intellectuals read with avidity the works of the important European scientific thinkers.

10. For a detailed account of the institutional development of science in the 1920s–1940s in Brazil, see Simon Schwartzman, *A formação da comunidade científica no Brasil* (São Paulo: Editora Nacional, 1979). For Peru, see Marcos Cueto, *Excelencia científica en la periferia: Actividades científicas e investigación biomédica en el Perú, 1890–1950* (Lima: Concyteec, 1989). For Argentina, José Babini, *Historia de la ciencia en la Argentina* (Buenos Aires: Ediciones Solar, 1986); Marcello Montserrat, "La introducción de la ciencia moderna en Argentina: El caso Gould," *Criterio* 44 (November 1971): 726–29; and Lewis Pyenson, *Cultural Imperialism and Exact Sciences—German Expansion Overseas, 1900–1930* (New York: Peter Lang, 1985). The latter book has very interesting material on Argentinian scientific institutions.

They embraced science as a form of progressive knowledge, as an alternative to the religious view of reality, and as a means of establishing a new form of cultural power. Evolution was adopted especially enthusiastically as a secular, materialist, modern view of the world.[11] Darwinism, which came to Latin America in the 1870s and 1880s from a variety of English, French, and German sources, and in forms that often departed considerably from Darwin's own ideas, was particularly resonant. The social Darwinisms taken up by intellectuals and scientists served as "meta-languages," providing rich, multivalent frameworks for the analysis of the history of the Latin American peoples and their destinies.[12] The new sciences were particularly attractive to the modern, secular, liberal intelligentsia, because they represented rational approaches to the natural and social world which were unencumbered by traditional religious considerations. As a result, evolution was initially associated with liberal and radical circles, rather than with the right. But evolutionism, like eugenics later, also had its darker side; it lent itself to racist formulations, and these formulations also became part of the intellectual baggage of the new scientific circles.

Of all the branches of science cultivated in Latin America, medicine was the most institutionally advanced and professionalized. Medical schools had been among the first scientifically oriented institutions to be established in Latin America. Throughout the nineteenth century, medical education, along with law, served as Latin American equivalents of, or substitutes for, the liberal arts degree;

11. On the impact of evolutionism and positivism in Latin America, see Charles A. Hale, "Political and Social Ideas in Latin America," in *The Cambridge History of Latin America*, ed. Leslie Bethell (Cambridge: Cambridge University Press, 1986), 4:382–414. On evolutionism in Argentina, see Marcelo Montserrat, "La presencia evolucionista en el positivismo argentino," *Quipu: Revista Latinoamericana de Historia de las Ciencias y la Tecnología* 3 (January–April 1986): 91–102; and Eduardo L. Ortiz, "La polémica del Darwinismo y la inserción de la ciencia en Argentina," *Actas II Congreso de la Sociedad Española de Historia de las Ciencias*, 1984, pp. 89–108. On Mexico, see Enrique Beltrán, "Alfredo Dugés y el transformismo," *Quipu: Revista Latinoamericana de Historia de las Ciencias y la Tecnología* 5 (January–April 1988): 49–58; and Roberto Moreno, "Mexico," in *The Comparative Reception of Darwinism*, ed. Thomas F. Glick (Chicago: University of Chicago Press, 1988), pp. 346–74. And on Brazil, see Terezinha Alves Ferreira Collichio, *Miranda Azevedo e o Darwinismo no Brasil* (São Paulo: Editores de Universidade de São Paulo, 1988).

12. On evolution as a "meta-language" see Julio Orione, "Florentino Ameghino y la influencia de Lamarck en la paleontología argentina del siglo XIX," *Quipu: Revista Latinoamericana de Historia de las Ciencias y la Tecnología* 4(3) (1987): 447–71.

many students attending medical school either failed to graduate or, once graduating, used their degrees for social advancement rather than as a means to professional practice. Medicine, then, was not a narrow, scientific, and technical profession but one connected to the larger social issues of the day. In the 1870s and 1880s in Brazil, for example, many physicians were republicans and Darwinists who actively participated in the movements for the abolition of slavery and the monarchy.

By the early twentieth century, medicine was beginning to become both more technical and scientific, and more expansive in its social role. This professionalization and expansion was largely a function of the generalized institutional growth of science that occurred throughout the region between roughly 1890 and 1930; more concretely it was a product of the revolution in medical science associated with bacteriology. For the first time, it appeared that doctors could actually begin to do something about the epidemic and endemic diseases that plagued urban and rural populations. As a result, "Pasteur" institutes dotted the institutional landscape of medicine by the early twentieth century.

In Brazil, a threatened epidemic of bubonic plague in 1899 led to the establishment of what became the federally funded Oswaldo Cruz Institute in Rio de Janiero. The extraordinary success of the public-health campaigns against smallpox, the bubonic plague, and yellow fever, led by the bacteriologist and director of the institute between 1903 and 1909, gave great cachet to the sanitation sciences. Oswaldo Cruz became a cultural hero among the elite, one of the first to be acclaimed for his role as a scientist. He went on to make the institute into a school of tropical medicine and as such the best-known center of biological research in Latin America at the time.[13] Cruz's career was matched by a number of other medical scientists who became, if not household names, at least well-known figures in Brazilian intellectual and political circles—Carlos Chagas, Artur Neiva, Henrique da Rocha Lima. A similar process of "pasteurization" of medicine occurred in several other countries of Latin America.

By the opening decades of the twentieth century, public health had thus become a politically accepted objective. The biological-en-

13. Details taken from chapter 5 of my book *Beginnings of Brazilian Science* [note 6].

gineering–technocratic approach to human populations which had long been familiar in Europe was beginning to emerge in Latin America; healthy and fit populations were seen as essential to material wealth, and the continued high rates of illness in the region a dreadful impediment to progress. Moreover, since medical education and public-health organizations were usually state-financed in Latin America, the state was viewed as a natural ally of doctors. The successes in bacteriology in Latin America stimulated the growth of a scientifically oriented professional and medical class that was increasingly visible and integrated into state and federal policy organizations.[14]

At the same time as expectations about the control of disease increased, the diseases most often associated with poverty—tuberculosis, venereal infections, alcoholism—pushed at the limits of medical knowledge and social expertise. They did not lend themselves easily to control by the new sciences of bacteriology and microbiology. The etiology of alcoholism was unknown, though it was clearly associated with poverty. But was poverty the cause or the result of alcoholism? The causative organism of syphilis had been discovered, and treatment was available in the drug Salvarsan, but the incidence of venereal disease remained alarmingly high throughout the continent. Tuberculosis dogged the lives of many poor people, thereby contributing a large share to national morbidity and mortality; yet moral and medical campaigns seemed hardly to dent the statistics. The continued high rates of mortality among the poor, especially children, were worrying to the elite because they challenged the ability of Latin American nations to follow the well-known prescription of the Argentinian statesman and educator J. B. Alberdi: "to govern is to populate."[15] How was Brazil to fill up its vast but empty spaces, or Argentina its pampas? How could these countries exploit their potentially large natural resources without healthy working populations?

Closely related to the issue of disease was that of the family itself, where all the problems of modernity seemed to many people to come together and threaten it with collapse. Old-fashioned and formally Catholic, middle-class Latin Americans venerated the tradi-

14. Ibid.
15. J. B. Alberdi, *Bases y puntos de partidos para la organización política de la República Argentina* (Buenos Aires: Librería de la Facultad de Juan Roldán, 1915).

tional family as the fundamental institution of the good society. That traditional family seemed increasingly at risk in the first decades of the twentieth century because of the growing presence of women in the workplace, new sexual mores that came with modernity and immigration, and the prostitution, illegitimacy, illegal abortions, and alcoholism that accompanied increasing industrialization, internal migration, urbanization, and immiseration. One answer to the dilemmas posed by a diseased body politic was to sanitize, moralize, and "eugenize" the family.[16] The focus on women and children within the family seemed natural enough, given that death from "weakness" and stillbirths accounted for 70 percent of the mortality of all newborn infants even in the medically advanced city of São Paulo.[17] Eugenics appealed, then, to an expanding medical class, eager to promote its role as specialists of the social life, and naively optimistic about its own power to do good. It was a class that, by the 1920s, was little given to revolutionary analyses of the economic, political, and racial roots of Latin America's social miseries.

Lastly, the emergence of eugenics in Latin America was conditioned by the region's racial ideologies. Brazilians, for instance, saw themselves as a racially mixed and largely dark-skinned people, the product of generations of crossings among Indians, Africans and Europeans. Concern about Brazil's racial makeup dated back to the first efforts at colonial rule by the Portuguese. And ever since the transfer of the Portuguese crown from Lisbon to Rio de Janeiro in 1808, race and race relations had been central to political-ideological debates about Brazilian capacity for development and the country's national destiny. Brazilian doubts about the country's racial identity had long been reinforced by racist interpretations of Brazil from abroad. Wilson Martins comments that Brazilians had a tendency to "live vicariously their own existence, as though it were a reflection in a mirror."[18] Intellectuals had to contend with the fact that, in text

16. Protoeugenic ideas predated the period of the eugenics movement in Brazil, as they did in other countries. See Dain Edward Borges, *The Family in Bahia, Brazil* (Stanford: Stanford University Press, 1992), on the decline of the traditional patriarchal family and some of the proposals put forward for its regeneration.

17. Robin L. Anderson, "Public Health and Public Healthiness: São Paulo, Brazil, 1876–1893," *Journal of the History of Medicine* 41 (1986): 293–307.

18. Wilson Martins, *Historia da inteligência brasileira*, 6 vols. (Rio de Janeiro: Editora da Universidade de São Paulo, 1915–1933), 5:6.

after European text, Brazil was held up as a prime example of the "degeneration" that occurred in a racially mixed, tropical nation. Henry Thomas Buckle, Benjamin Kidd, Georges Vacher de Lapouge, Gustave Le Bon, the Count de Gobineau, and various social Darwinists were widely quoted for their theories of Negro inferiority, mulatto degeneration, and tropical decay. From the United States the message was the same; as evidence that "halfbreeds" could not produce a high civilization, anthropologists pointed to Latin Americans, who, they claimed, were now "paying for their racial liberality."[19] According to U.S. thinkers, the "promiscuous" crossings that had occurred in much of Latin America had produced a degenerate, unstable people incapable of progressive development.

To a large extent the educated classes of Latin America shared the misgivings of the Europeans. They wished to be white and feared they were not. For this reason, encouragement of European immigration had by the end of the nineteenth century become national policy in many of the countries of Latin America. White immigrant labor, it was believed, would contribute to a more progressive society and would improve a country's image as a potentially white nation. The role of science in the debate about race and destiny was a further and complicating factor. By the early twentieth century, science everywhere had emerged as a critical component of cultural interpretation and its racism had also intensified—whether in medicine, psychiatry, biology, anthropology, or the social sciences. In Latin America, science therefore proved to be a two-edged sword. On the one hand, intellectuals saw science as progressive and liberating, offering authoritative new tools—intellectual and practical—for effecting a way out of their countries' supposed backwardness. On the other hand, science was increasingly allied to racism.

In Brazil, for instance, the themes of tropical and racial degeneration run through medical, bacteriological, and social writings from the early nineteenth century until well into the 1930s, the period of the revisionist theories of the sociologist Gilberto Freyre. Especially following abolition in 1888, science was increasingly used, as it had been in Europe since the Enlightenment, to define how much "nature" would limit the social and political equality of blacks and mulattoes in the new republic. Raimundo Nina Rodrigues, the founder

19. George W. Stocking, Jr., *Race, Culture, and Evolution: Essays in the History of Anthropology* (New York: Free Press, 1968), p. 50.

of the new scientific anthropology in Brazil in the 1890s, an anthropology that centered around the problem of race and that utilized all the new techniques of anthropometry, was almost as pessimistic in his outlook as Brazil's severest critics. His anthropological studies revealed to him not a white, "civilized" nation-in-the-making but a complicated, multiracial, heterogeneous country that had forged no single, stable ethnic type and whose foreseeable future was ethnically black.[20] Euclides da Cunha's classic work of social analysis, *Rebellion in the Backlands* (1902), which recounted the story of an armed revolt by the racially mixed *sertanejos* of Canudos in the poverty-stricken northeastern region of Brazil, synthesized the sciences of his day to argue that "miscegenation, in addition to obliterating the pre-eminent qualities of the higher race, serves to stimulate the revival of the primitive attributes of the lower; so that the mestizo—a hyphen between races, a brief individual existence into which are compressed age-old forces—is almost always an unbalanced type."[21] Given these circumstances and ideological inflections, eugenics, by definition the science of "racial improvement," could easily appeal to intellectuals and professionals convinced of the power of science to create "order and progress" (the motto of the Brazilian republic) and troubled by the racial makeup of their country.

The Institutionalization of Eugenics in Brazil

Although in some senses the social, economic, and ideological changes described here can be said to have created needs and demands that could be met by a program of eugenics, the development of that program required concrete institutional mediations.[22]

In Brazil, these mediations were provided largely by physicians, in an association between medicine and eugenics typical of Latin

20. Raimundo Nina Rodrigues, *As raças humanas e a responsibilidade no Brasil*, ed. Afrânio Peixoto (1894; Rio de Janeiro: Editora Nacional, 1938). Nina Rodrigues's work indicates a shift in the 1890s from environmentalist explanations of Brazil's condition toward more racist ones.

21. Euclides da Cunha, *Rebellion in the Backlands [Os sertões]*, trans. Samuel Putnam (1902; Chicago: Chicago University Press, 1944), p. 85.

22. This point was made by William Bynum in another context (a discussion of the emergence of the modern asylum); see *The Anatomy of Madness: Essays in the History of Psychiatry*, vol. 1: *People and Ideas*, ed. W. F. Bynum, Roy Porter, and Michael Shepherd (London: Tavistock Publications, 1985), pp. 7–8.

American eugenics as a whole. Physicians, together with lawyers, formed the largest of the professional groups in the region, and a medical education was the normal—often the only—route to scientific knowledge. Although eugenics had other advocates—indeed, eugenic language circulated in literary and political circles on the left and right—eugenics in Latin America was largely an "expert" phenomenon with conservative-reformist tendencies.

In late 1917, right at the time when strikes shut down the city of São Paulo, the capital of the most powerful state in the Brazilian republic, Renato Kehl, a young graduate in pharmacy and medicine, called a meeting of doctors to discuss the proposed revisions of the nation's civil marriage code, which would allow consanguineous marriages for the first time.[23] Most doctors opposed such marriages for religious or medical reasons. Kehl took the opportunity of the meeting to link human marriage explicitly to Galton's new science of eugenics. After the meeting, Kehl sent a circular to city and state physicians, proposing the creation of a new scientific society devoted specifically to the new eugenics and inviting his colleagues' participation. On January 25, 1918, the São Paulo Eugenics Society (Sociedade Eugénica de São Paulo) was born. Its founding represented the first step in the organized history of eugenics in Latin America and the beginning of a more or less continuous involvement by Latin Americans in eugenics from 1918 to the 1940s.[24]

The society's membership numbered 140, thus comparing favorably with the size of the French Eugenics Society (which at its peak had only just over a hundred members).[25] The size of a eugenics society anywhere was less important than the prominence of its members, and perhaps even less so in Brazil, where the educated class was very small by European standards. In its brief existence the São Paulo Eugenics Society attracted the attention of the medical elite of the city and nearby towns.[26] Of the members, only two were listed without the title "Dr.," which in Brazil usually (though not

23. E.g., marriages between uncles and nieces.
24. Renato Kehl, "The First Eugenics Movement in Brazil," *Boletim de Eugenía* 3(28) (1931): 35–36.
25. William Schneider, "Toward the Improvement of the Human Race: The History of Eugenics in France," *Journal of Modern History* 54 (June 1982): 277.
26. Joseph Love, in *São Paulo in the Brazilian Federation (1889–1937)* (Stanford: Stanford University Press, 1980), p. 154, points to the small size of the political elite between 1889 and 1937, naming only 263 individuals. The professional (e.g., medical, engineering) class was much larger.

always) signified graduation from either medical or law school. In fact, almost all the members were physicians.[27] The society had no women members, and only eighteen members from outside the state. In addition, the Argentine doctor Victor Delfino, who was on the brink of starting a eugenics society in Buenos Aires, and Carlos Enrique Paz Soldán, the Peruvian pioneer of "social medicine" (and later a prolific medical activist), were named as corresponding members.

The society sought to project itself beyond the boundaries of the state of São Paulo by asking Belisário Penna, a well-known advocate of sanitation based in Rio de Janeiro, to serve as one of three honorary vice presidents. The actual president was the physician Arnaldo Vieira de Carvalho, director of São Paulo's new medical school, which had been founded in 1913 and stood for all that was advanced in medical education at that time in Brazil. Among the society's more important members were Vital Brasil, the bacteriologist and director of the Butantã Institute (the well-known snake-serum research institute); Artur Neiva, a microbiologist from the Oswaldo Cruz Institute in Rio who had come to São Paulo to head and remodel the state's sanitation services; Luís Pereira Barreto, the Paulista medical writer and positivist; Antônio Austregesilo, psychiatrist and professor at the Rio Medical School; and the young Fernando de Azevedo, who would later go on to a distinguished career in education at the University of São Paulo, founded in the 1930s. Juliano Moreira, the most important mental hygienist in Brazil and the director of Brazil's National Mental Asylum in Rio de Janeiro, sent a letter of congratulation to the society and advised it of his own eugenical efforts in the field of mental hygiene.[28]

The São Paulo Eugenics Society had an initial success, holding regular meetings in the hall of the Santa Casa de Misericordia, the traditional meetingplace of the state's most important scientific group, the Medical and Surgical Society. From the beginning the society defined itself as a learned, scientific, professional organization from which would flow scientific studies, conferences, and pro-

27. Although "Dr." was also used as a courtesy title for prominent individuals who were not actually graduates of medicine or law, in the professional medical context in which eugenics appeared the title "Dr." in fact signified professional qualifications; nondoctors were indicated as "Senhor" (Mr.).

28. Details about the scientific careers of many of these individuals can be found in Stepan, *Beginnings of Brazilian Science* [note 6], passim.

paganda on the physical and moral strengthening of the Brazilian "race."[29] In fact, the society, despite its distinguished roster of medical scientists—most of them clinicians—carried out no research. Its main function was to propagandize the idea of eugenics and to introduce a new language into Brazilian debate. Traditional medical themes—alcoholism, venereal diseases, degeneration, fertility, natality, tuberculosis—were linked to the "purification" and eugenization of the nation.

The meetings of the society were organized by Kehl, who was to remain the chief spokesman for eugenics in Brazil and whose whole life was henceforth to be identified with the movement. Kehl's position as secretary allowed him to orchestrate the meetings in directions congenial to his view of eugenics. He reminded the members of the advances made in eugenics in Europe and of the need for Brazil to join the advanced nations in studying heredity, evolution, and the influences of the environment, economic conditions, legislation, customs, and habits on the health of people. He assured his listeners that eugenics was not a utopian fantasy but a reality of modern scientific nations.[30]

In addition to its regular sessions, the society organized several talks and conferences that brought eugenics into the public arena; for instance, Rubião Meira lectured on "factors of degeneration in our race and the means of combating them"; Kehl addressed the Young Men's Christian Association. Many of these talks were reprinted in a volume published by the society in 1919 as the *Annals of Eugenics*. The small size of the elite and the close contacts between journalism and medicine gave eugenics a hearing in the daily and weekly press. The reaction was highly favorable; eugenics was greeted as a new science capable of ushering in a new social order through the medical perfecting of the human race.[31]

Despite initial enthusiasm, however, the São Paulo Eugenics Society came to an end in late 1919, unable to survive Carvalho's death that year and Kehl's own departure for Rio de Janeiro. With Kehl's move the locus of eugenics passed northeast to the federal capital of Rio de Janeiro. There Kehl kept the interest in eugenics alive with numerous pamphlets, books, and lectures, many of which were re-

29. *Annães de eugenia* (São Paulo: Revista do Brasil, 1919), p. 35.
30. As reported later by Kehl in *Lições de eugenia* [note 3], pp. 15–27.
31. *Annães de eugenia* [note 29], pp. 15–16.

ported in the medical press and daily newspapers. By 1947 Kehl had published no fewer than twenty-six books, many of which the press reviewed favorably. In addition to Kehl's writings, Belisário Penna's *The Army and Sanitation* (1920) was part of the early eugenics effort, as was J. B. Monteiro Lobato's *The Vital Problem* (1918), which was published jointly by the São Paulo Eugenics Society and the Pro-Sanitation League (Liga Pro-Saneamento do Brasil). In his multivolume study of Brazilian writing, Wilson Martins refers to a veritable stream of works on eugenics and related themes in the 1920s and 1930s, expressing a nostalgia for hygiene and "purification."[32] As the eugenic creed won new converts, the language of eugenics began to infuse scientific discussions of health. Improvement was now discussed in terms of "eugenic" and "dysgenic" factors, fitness and unfitness, and hereditary "taras" (defects). Penna's 1918 book, *The Sanitation of Brazil*, had been devoid of eugenic language; his new book of 1920, based on a series of lectures to the Military Club of Rio and published as *The Army and Sanitation*, had the same theme—the disgraceful state of sanitation in Brazil—but now the problem was presented as that of the hereditary degeneration of the Brazilian people and the need for a eugenic solution.

Although initally Kehl was unable to organize a new society devoted specifically to eugenics in the federal capital, eugenics found a place for itself within the field of mental hygiene—an association between eugenics and psychiatry repeated in several other Latin American countries.[33] Through this association, eugenics became linked to the problems of criminality, juvenile delinquency, and prostitution—to the social "pathologies" of the poor, and, in the case of Brazil, of the racially mixed and dark population. Mental hygiene was defined as a preventive form of psychiatric medicine which of necessity extended the scope of the doctor beyond the

32. Martins, *Historia da inteligência brasileira* [note 18], 6:263. According to a bibliography of eugenics prepared by Kehl, in *Aparas eugénicas: Sexo e civilização* (Rio de Janeiro: Francisco Alves, 1933), pp. 261–71, between 1897 and 1933 seventy-four important publications on eugenics appeared in Brazil; these included twenty-four undergraduate medical theses from the Faculty of Medicine in Rio de Janeiro. In fact, Kehl underrepresented the production of eugenics literature in Brazil by omitting many books, pamphlets, and articles that did not fit his own definition of eugenics—for instance, some of the writings of his critic Dr. Octavio Domingues. See Chapter 3 of this book for an explanation.

33. In Peru, for example, a eugenics section was created within the League of Mental Hygiene in the 1930s.

walls of the asylum and into everyday life in the home, the streets, and the schools. Mental hygiene, though representing itself as a modern and innovative approach to insanity and crime, was, in the Latin American context, deeply tinged with hereditarianism, especially the extreme hereditarianism of the Italian criminologist Cesare Lombroso.[34] Eugenically oriented mental hygiene can be seen as a further elaboration and "modernization" of Lombroso's teaching that criminal traits are inherited.

The psychiatrist Gustavo Reidel founded the new League of Mental Hygiene (Liga de Higiene Mental) in 1922 in Rio in order to realize a practical program of mental prophylaxis, with a focus on the mentally "deficient," disturbed, and delinquent individuals who, the doctors believed, were hereditarily prone to commit crimes and therefore needed to be identified, diagnosed, and, if necessary, segregated from the rest of the population for purposes of "restraint" and treatment. Like the U.S. psychiatrists whom the mental hygienists wished to emulate, the league's members considered themselves progressives in the sense of being oriented toward individual psychiatric treatment and, in the case of the criminally insane, toward the treatment of the criminal person rather than the crime.[35] The League of Mental Hygiene represented itself, therefore, as a professional and scientific organization associated with advanced psychiatry in the rest of the world.[36]

34. On Lombroso, see Robert A. Nye, *Crime, Madness, and Politics in Modern France: The Medical Concept of National Decline* (Princeton, N.J.: Princeton University Press, 1984), chap. 4, and Daniel Pick, "The Faces of Anarchy: Lombroso and the Politics of Criminal Science in Post-Unification Italy," *History Workshop* 21 (Spring 1986): 60–86. Lombroso's influence, and more generally that of the Italian school of criminology, is apparent in the many references to Lombroso in Latin American anthropological and criminological writing. To my knowledge, however, this influence has yet to be studied.

35. For a history of the mental-hygiene movement in the United States, see Gerald N. Grob, *Mental Illness and American Society, 1875–1940* (Princeton, N.J.: Princeton University Press, 1983), chap. 6. Grob describes in some detail the involvement of the mental-hygiene movement with eugenics, especially eugenic sterilization.

36. David J. Rothman, in *Conscience and Convenience: The Asylum and Its Alternatives in Progressive America* (Boston: Little, Brown, 1980), esp. pp. 5–6, discusses the confused motives and the often sad consequences of "progressive" thought on the mentally ill in the early twentieth century in the United States. The Brazilians consciously modeled themselves on their North American counterparts. A short account of psychiatry in Brazil in the 1930s is found in Jurandir Freire Costa, *História de psiquiatria no Brasil: Um corto ideología* (Rio de Janeiro: Editora Documentário, 1976). A history of the most important mental asylum in São Paulo and its connec-

The league quickly established itself in the city, with more than 120 members drawn from the staffs of the state and municipal mental asylums and reformatories. The league organized ten permanent committees and held regular monthly meetings. Although its subventions from the municipality of Rio and the federal government were not always adequate or secure, the league enjoyed considerable success as one of the more prominent of the scientifically oriented societies of the federal capital.[37] Eugenics was part of the league's program from the start; its statutes declared its purpose was to "realize a program of mental hygiene and eugenics in individual, school, professional and social life."[38] But the league's emphasis on eugenics intensified over the years as a new generation of psychiatrists, led by Ernani Lopes (who became president in 1929), took over the organization. The league also managed to get official sanction for its activities; for instance, in 1927 a new law of assistance to the mentally ill was introduced which was sponsored by Afrânio Peixoto, a member of the league; this law gave to psychiatrists and mental hygienists the power to commit the mentally ill to asylums and also expanded dispensaries and local consulting services in the cities. To signify the mental improvement of the race, the psychiatrists coined a new term, "euphrenia."[39]

Kehl became active in the league by 1925. By 1929 the league's membership included many of the more prominent medical scientists of the city, such as Juliano Moreira, director of the National Mental Asylum; Miguel Couto, president of the National Academy of Medicine and Rio's leading clinician; Fernando Magalhães, professor of gynecology and obstetrics at the Rio Medical School; Carlos Chagas, discoverer of "Chagas" disease (*Trypanosomiasis americana*) and director of both the Oswaldo Cruz Institute and the federal Department of Public Health; Edgar Roquette-Pinto, director of the National Museum in Rio; the hygienist and pioneer of legal medicine Afrânio Peixoto; and the psychiatrists Henrique Roxo

---

tions to the São Paulo League of Mental Hygiene is Maria Clementina Pereira Cunha's *O espelho do mundo: Juquery, a história de um asilo* (Rio de Janeiro: Paz e Terra, 1986).

37. Details of the league's history can be traced in its journal, the *Archivos Brasileiros de Hygiene Mental* (hereafter *ABHM*).

38. *ABHM* 2(2) (1929): 39–47, and 13(1) (1941): 91–95.

39. *ABHM* 5(2) (1932):3; on the law, see Pereira Cunha, *O espelho do mundo* [note 36], p. 170.

and Antônio Austregesilo. In 1929 the league resumed publication of its journal, the *Brazilian Archives of Mental Hygiene*, which had been interrupted after its first issue in 1925. It intensified its agitation against alcoholism, clarifying in the media its connection to "racial degeneration."

Another venue for eugenics in Brazil was legal medicine, a growing Latin American specialization seeking to find institutional solidity and a clearly defined role. By the second decade of the twentieth century, several professorial chairs and institutes in legal medicine had been established, usually within existing medical faculties (many of the professors were in fact jurists rather than doctors). In legal medicine the problems of crime and responsibility became closely linked in the minds of doctors to the racial issue and eugenics. Afrânio Peixoto wrote widely on eugenic themes, promoting the use of eugenics in police work and in reducing hereditary criminality, and generally advocating cooperation between the legal and medical professions.[40] Meanwhile, eugenics also made its appearance in discussions at the National Academy of Medicine, where Miguel Couto made eugenics and immigration his special topic.[41] At the National Museum, Roquette-Pinto produced a book in 1927 with a long chapter on the "laws of eugenics" and their anthropological significance for Brazil.[42]

These various strands of eugenics came together in July 1929 in the most important public manifestation of Brazilian eugenics of the 1920s, the First Brazilian Eugenics Congress. The occasion for the congress was the centennial celebration of the founding of the National Academy of Medicine. With Roquette-Pinto presiding, the week-long congress was attended by some two hundred professionals, including medical clinicians, officials from the state psychiatric and sanitation institutions and services, journalists, and several federal deputies representing various political viewpoints. Delegates from Argentina, Peru, Chile, and Paraguay were also present, including Paz Soldán, whose 1916 pamphlet *A National Program of Sanitary Politics* had long been claimed by the Brazilians as a fundamental eugenics text.[43]

40. See, e.g., Afrânio Peixoto's *Criminología* (São Paulo: Editora Nacional, 1933).

41. *Boletim da Academia Nacional de Medicina* 96(2) (1923): 33–34.

42. Edgar Roquette-Pinto, *Seixos rolados (Estudos brasileiros)* (Rio de Janeiro: n.p., 1927).

43. *Brasil-Médico* 43 (1929): 842–45 gives a good account of the congress.

The congress's themes were broad indeed—marriage and eugenics, eugenic education, the protection of "nationality," racial types and eugenics, the importance of genealogical archives, Japanese immigration, antivenereal campaigns, intoxicants and eugenics, the treatment of the mentally ill, sex education, and the protection of infants and mothers. The participants passed several resolutions, the most controversial being a call for a national immigration law to restrict entry into Brazil to those individuals deemed eugenically "sound" on the basis of some kind of medical test.

The success of the congress and the publicity it received in the daily and medical press suggested that eugenics was about to enter a new phase of activity. Already in January 1929, Kehl had begun publishing a monthly journal, the *Bulletin of Eugenics*.[44] Two years later, in the so-called Revolution of 1930, the foundations of the First Republic were thrown in question. A period of political disturbance and agitation ensued which, in conjunction with the economic hardships caused by the world depression, helped to expand the political and ideological space for eugenic propaganda. The eugenic ideal of a rationally managed, medically purified society transcending class conflicts was shared by other nationalistic, antidemocratic, and organic statist ideologies that flourished in the period. The ever energetic Kehl seized the political opportunity to create the Central Brazilian Commission of Eugenics to promote eugenics at the national level and raise the issue of immigration as a pressing national-medical issue. In 1933, the eugenists turned their attention to lobbying the newly elected members of the Constituent Assembly, which had a wide mandate to reexamine aspects of Brazilian politics. The eugenists were remarkably successful in inserting eugenics into the new immigration-restriction law and legislation concerning marriage.[45] The League of Mental Hygiene also revived its *Archives* and intensified its eugenics work, as can be seen from its numerous editorials calling for an officially endorsed antialcohol campaign and immigration selection, and in the creation of its first Infants Euphrenic Clinic.[46]

44. The journal *Boletim de Eugenia* appeared as a separate section within the medical journal *Medicamenta* but carried its own title and editorial board. I refer to it in this book under its own name.
45. For a discussion, see Chapters 3 and 4.
46. *ABHM* 7(1) (1934): 65.

Eugenics in Spanish America

The feeling that the moment was ripe for eugenics was confirmed by the emergence of eugenics in other countries. Hardly a single area in Latin America had in fact remained completely untouched by eugenics by the 1930s. Obviously, the social and political conditions of Latin American nations varied greatly. Nevertheless, their eugenics societies and activities followed in most respects the pattern already described for Brazil—they were led by medical doctors in obstetrics, child health, and mental hygiene, and their goals were to propagandize, and apply, the new science of eugenics rather than to carry out research in heredity and health. Two of the most important eugenics associations in the hemisphere were founded in this period: the Mexican Eugenics Society for the Improvement of Race (Sociedad Eugénica Mexicana para el Mejoramiento de la Raza) and the Argentine Association of Biotypology, Eugenics, and Social Medicine (Associación Argentina de Biotipología, Eugenesia y Medicina Social). Both enjoyed the membership of some of the well-known medical scientists of the times, regular meetings (weekly at first in the Mexican case), their own journals, the confidence of their professional peers, and on occasion political prominence.

Mexican eugenics was one of the most interesting of our cases because of its revolutionary setting. The revolution in Mexico between 1910 and 1920 was the first of the profound social and political upheavals that marked the twentieth century; it was devastating in the scale of its violence. The deaths and dislocations caused by the war and the staggering problems of poverty and sickness, combined with the growing nationalism of the revolutionary state, provided the setting for the appeal to eugenics. Ideologically, the revolution's socialism, anticlericism, and materialism made Mexico receptive to new developments in science and social thought. Darwinian ideas were familiar, and many Mexican biologists, such as Alfonso L. Herrera, were convinced evolutionists and materialists who believed deeply in the power of science to improve the human lot.[47] Mexico was not an immigrant society but an "Indian" and mestizo one; decades of debate about how the Indian population would become integrated into the national whole and how the health of the poor could

47. For a study of the reception of Darwin in Mexico, see Moreno, "Mexico," and Beltrán, "Alfredo Dugés y el transformismo" [note 11].

be improved now converged on eugenics. A pamphlet on "stirpiculture" by a Mexican, Fortuno Hernández, appeared in 1910. According to one account, the first public notice of eugenics occurred the
next year, when the work of the British eugenist Caleb Saleeby on
what he called "eugenical feminism" attracted attention.[48] In 1921
Herrera predicted that laboratory science would one day produce a
race of supermen who would "populate the earth with a new and
perfect humanity."[49] Left-wing, radical, and socialist strands in eugenics existed in several European countries (e.g., Russia and Germany in the 1920s), so the adoption of eugenics by socialist circles in
Mexico was therefore not unique; socialists' endorsement prevented
eugenics from becoming a preserve of the right.

By the 1920s eugenics had been incorporated into Mexican med-
ico-social debates. As the phrase "eugenical feminism" suggests,
some of these debates involved women and reproductive health.
Women, some of them feminists, were actively involved in eugenics
in Germany and elsewhere in the 1920s because of their concern
with healthy motherhood and healthy babies and their worries about
high rates of infant and maternal morbidity. In most Latin American
countries, as we shall see, feminism as an idea and a movement was
slow to develop. Where it did it was severely attacked as unnatural;
in the circumstances, a feminist eugenics was very much a minority
position.[50] In Mexico in 1921, however, the Mexican Congress of
the Child raised eugenic and sexual issues; it even voted in favor of
sterilization of criminals—a harbinger of the more extreme eugenics
that would eventually surface in Mexico.[51] By 1929 the new Mexi-

48. Fortuno Hernández, *Higiene de la especie: Breves consideraciones sobre la stir-
picultura humana* (Mexico City: Bouligny e Schmidt, 1910). Alfredo Saavedra in "Lo
'eugénico' anunciado por primera vez en México," *Acción Médica* (September 1956):
16–17, refers to an article in *El Diario* in 1911 on Saleeby's idea that a eugenics
program would protect women from venereal and other damaging factors that could
affect the health of their offspring; Saleeby believed such a program would be "feminist."

49. The quotation is found in Herrera's footnote to Israel Castellanos's *Plasmogenia* (Havana: Rambla, Bouza, 1921), p. 124. "Plasmogenesis" was Herrera's
word for the experimental, materialist science of the phenomena associated with
protoplasm and therefore life.

50. I take up the themes of reproduction, gender, and eugenics in Chapter 4.

51. The first congress [Congreso del Niño] was followed by a second in 1923. On
eugenics at the congresses, see the references in Alfredo Saavedra M., "Lo que México ha publicado acerca de eugenesia," in Ateneo Nacional de Ciencias y Artes,
Primer Congreso Bibliográfico Mexicano (Mexico City: DAPP, 1937), pp. 103–25.

can Society of Puericulture (Sociedad Mexicana de Puericultura) that formed in Mexico City had created a eugenics section, where issues of heredity, disease, infantile sexuality, sex education, and birth control—radical ideas for their time and place—were discussed in relation to the care of the child.

The lack of more solid institutional development of eugenics before the 1930s in Mexico was due in part to the political and social uncertainties caused by the revolution itself, the consequent difficulties experienced by scientists, and ideological clashes over religion.[52] It was not until the early 1930s, in a moment of relative conservatism within the revolution and institutional consolidation of the revolution's political and state structures, that eugenics made an independent appearance in Mexico. In the autumn of 1931 a group of doctors and scientifically minded reformers, many of whom had been active in public health and puericulture, organized the Mexican Eugenics Society in the federal capital. Quickly making up for lost time, the 130-odd members held some thirty-one sessions by October of that year alone. The society was connected to several of the state governments of the Mexican Republic, with representatives from state public-health departments as well as the federal Department of Public Health.[53] Several well-known biologists were associated with the society in the 1930s, including Fernando Ocaranza, who played an active role, and José Rulfo, who is credited with being the first Mexican scientist to introduce modern experimental Mendelian genetics in Mexico in the late 1930s and early 1940s.

By May 1932 the society had set up a permanent technical commission to respond to requests for information and advice, and by August its *Bulletin* began publication (later to change its name to *Eugenics*). In February the following year, the permanent secretary and dominating figure in the eugenics movement, Alfredo Saavedra, drew up a Mexican Code of Eugenics. By this time the national

52. Herrera describes some of these difficulties in his short history of biology in Mexico, *La biología en México durante un siglo* (Mexico City: El Democrata, 1921). The history of health policies in the 1920s and 1930s and their connection to other social and political agendas of the revolution sorely need analysis.

53. A brief history of the society appeared in an editorial in the journal *Eugenesia* new ser. 1 (March 1940): 1–6. This journal started as the *Boletín de la Sociedad Eugénica Mexicana* and changed its name to *Eugenesia* in December 1931. Further details about the Mexican Eugenics Society are drawn from Alfredo Saavedra, *México en la educación sexual (de 1860 a 1959)* (Mexico City: Costa-Amic, 1967), and from his article "Lo que México ha publicado acerca de eugenesia" [note 51].

press had given eugenics wide, if stormy, publicity by announcing the extensive program of eugenically oriented sex education the society had proposed to the national government, following a request from the National Block of Revolutionary Women.[54]

The Argentine Association of Biotypology, Eugenics, and Social Medicine in Buenos Aires was founded in 1932 in very different political circumstances. On a per capita basis, Argentina was a rich country, a fact that drew to its shores millions of immigrants looking to improve their lot in life. It also had a large medical profession, which performed very creditably in controlling epidemic and endemic diseases at a time of a huge influx of very poor people from Europe; the improvement in mortality and morbidity rates made Buenos Aires if anything ahead of New York in health statistics.

As in Brazil and Mexico, eugenic ideas were picked up early, long before the Great War. In Argentina, eugenics was first associated with the secular and modern left-wing and anarchist groups which played such an important part in Argentine cultural and political life in the first two decades of the twentieth century. In 1909, for example, Argentina's Emilio Coni, the socialist physician who published widely on sanitation, attended a medical congress in Chile in 1909 and embarrassed his fellow Argentinian physicians by discussing birth control and eugenic sterilization. Like many socialists, Coni viewed eugenic legislation on procreation as a progressive and necessary part of medical sanitation.[55] Eugenics was also a feature of psychiatric and criminological societies and progressive reform circles.

The first move toward the concretization of a eugenics society occurred in 1912, when the physician Victor Delfino attended the First International Congress of Eugenics in London (the only Latin American to do so, as far as I have been able to establish) and reported back on the results of the debates about eugenics then taking place in the advanced centers of science. Delfino founded the Argen-

54. See Saavedra, *México en la educación sexual* [note 53], p. 34.

55. Emilio Coni, "Frecuencia y profilaxis de las enfermedades venéreas en la América Latina," in *Trabajos del Cuarto Congreso Científico* (I Panamericana) (Santiago: Imprenta Barcelona, 1909), 1:391–433. References to eugenics can also be found in the anarchist journal *La Protesta* in the same period, as well as in various journals of psychiatry and criminology. Another interesting anarchist and eugenist was Georg Friedrich Nicolai, a German who came to Argentina after his opposition to World War I had led to his explusion from his country; see Wolf Zuelzer, *The Nicolai Case: A Biography* (Detroit: Wayne State University Press, 1982).

tine Eugenics Society in 1918. His activities reflected a reorientation of eugenics in much more conservative and racist directions; this shift intensified during the economic crisis that spanned the war years, a crisis that tested the faith of the secular and professional classes in the inevitability of Argentinian progress. Growing worries about national identity and the disturbances to national culture and mores caused by "foreign" customs and peoples made immigration and race salient issues. In his pronouncements, Delfino connected eugenics to the need for national purification and above all to immigration controls. But the eugenics committee and society Delfino founded, in 1914 and 1918 respectively, and the Argentine League of Social Prophylaxis led by Alfredo Verano in the 1920s, though important indicators of the direction eugenics was taking in Argentina, were only preludes to the more fully developed eugenic efforts in the 1930s, yet another period of economic crisis.[56]

The Argentine Association of Biotypology, Eugenics, and Social Medicine, established in 1932 in Buenos Aires, came into existence in a very conservative, even reactionary moment of Argentinian history; its founding signaled a definitive shift in the ideology of eugenics in the country from the left to the right. Already in the 1920s, as new cultural mores, democratic demands, and labor unrest challenged the traditional political system, the elites had hardened their attitudes toward immigration. They expressed cultural nostalgia for their "hispanic" past and resisted various classes of immigrants as putative carriers of strange cultural mores and unfamiliar diseases. Politically, the long period of dominance by the Radical party, which in the 1920s had led to the opening up of society and politics to some of the demands of the middle class and immigrant groups, came to an end in a military coup in 1930. The events signaled the beginning of an era of conservatism that lasted until 1943, the year Juan Perón appeared on the political scene. The 1930s were marked by weak political parties, fraudulent elections, antiforeign sentiment, and hostility to "alien" peoples and cultural practices. Old and new nationalisms came together in a shared dislike of liberalism, democracy, and foreign capital. The church, whose influence in education and in its traditional sphere of marriage had been limited by the

56. These early initiatives are analyzed in Chapters 3 and 5. On the early uses of eugenic ideas and language, see Eduardo Zimmerman, "Racial Ideas and Social Reform in Argentina" (Oxford: unpublished paper, 1989).

secular legislation introduced in the second half of the nineteenth century, began to stage a comeback, seeking to extend its role among the new urban masses and among the elite. The Argentine Catholic Action (founded in 1928) had by the mid-1930s become a vehicle for expressing antidemocratic, even profascist sentiment.[57]

The Association of Biotypology, founded in this moment of reaction, was unusual in being linked directly to a peculiar Italian science, "biotypology." This was perhaps the most significant of all the new eugenics societies in Latin America in the scale of its ambition and in its distinctive scientific character. The cultural influence of Italy was much greater in Argentina than in Brazil (where Italians also settled in large numbers), owing to the larger size of the middle class in Argentina and the more open political and educational system.

The direct inspiration for the association was the visit to the country of the Genoese scientist and originator of the word "biotypology," Nicola Pende (called Nicolás in Spanish) in 1930. The central idea of biotypology was that human populations could be divided into distinct types with their own characteristic illnesses and psychological makeup. Biotypology was concerned not only with the classification of individuals into their correct types but with the control of development—physical, psychic, and sexual—so that "normality" could be ensured and abnormalities be prevented. Pende believed that by means of an inventory of human biotypes in a population the biological resources of a nation could be harnessed efficiently to the goals of the state. Such an endeavor, said Pende, was of vital concern to the fascists and the work of Mussolini.

In Argentina, biotypology was explicitly linked to eugenics, a link that provided an opportunity to bring together a variety of physicians long interested in maternity, child health, and heredity and that directed their attention to the steps that could be taken to improve the "biotypes" of the Argentinian population by the study and control of its "orthogenetic" development. Gender and racial considerations figured prominently in this eugenics. The Argentine association quickly became one of the largest medical associations in the country, incorporating into its organization many figures from

57. Nestor T. Azua, *Los católicos argentinos: Su experiencia política y social* (Buenos Aires: Editorial Clarentiana, 1984).

past eugenic efforts as well as new recruits.[58] Of all the eugenics organizations in the region it had the most substantial institutional representation, with its own school for training experts in the diagnostic methods of biotypology and a polyclinic for evaluation and treatment. The latter opened ceremoniously in 1933 in the presence of the president of the republic, General Agustín P. Justo.

In addition to the growth of eugenics nationally, eugenics was becoming a Pan American affair. The first Pan American Conference of Eugenics and Homiculture, held in 1927, was the occasion for a debate on a proposed Pan American Code of Eugenics; a second conference followed in Buenos Aires in 1934. In the following year the Latin International Federation of Eugenics Societies was organized in Mexico City, with representation not only from Latin America but also from several European countries.[59] The two most significant Peruvian celebrations of eugenics were held even later, in 1939 and 1943.[60] Legislatively, the period also witnessed the passage of a variety of eugenic laws regulating race and marriage, as we shall see.[61] An Argentine physician commented in 1943 that everything seemed to point to the "present hour" as the "hour of eugenics."[62]

The renewed energy in Brazilian eugenics in the 1930s, the formation of new eugenics institutions in Argentina, Mexico, and elsewhere, and the persistence of eugenics into the 1940s and even later raise some interesting questions concerning the continuities and discontinuities in the history of eugenics and the meanings attached to

58. Victor Delfino's Argentine Eugenics Society [Sociedad Eugénica Argentina] apparently came to an end sometime in the 1920s. An explanation of the meaning of biotypology and its connection to eugenics was given by one of the leading lights of the new organization, Dr. Artur R. Rossi, in his "Curso sintético de medicina constitucional y biotipología: Herencia y constitución," *Anales de Biotipología, Eugenesia y Medicina Social* (hereafter *ABEMS*) 1 (May 1, 1933): 12–14; see also Dr. Arturo León López, "Eugenesia," *ABEMS* 1 (May 15, 1933): 17–18. Further discussion of biotypology and eugenics is found in Chapters 3, 4, and 5.

59. A discussion and analysis of the Pan American and Latin federations is found in Chapter 6.

60. Dr. Guillermo Fernandez Dávila, "La obra eugenésica en el Perú," *Primera Jornada Peruana de Eugenesia* (Lima: n.p., 1940), pp. 46–52, and Carlos A. Banbarén, "La eugenesia en América," *Eugenesia* new ser. 1 (March 1940): 7–10.

61. Dr. Enrique Díaz de Guijarro, "La eugenesia y la reciente legislación del matrimonio en América Latina," *Crónica Médica* 61 (1944): 230–36, 282–94. See Chapter 4.

62. Juan Pou Orfila, "Reflexiones sobre la eugenesia en América Latina," *Obstetricia y Ginecología Latino-Americana* (Buenos Aires) 1(1) (1943): 50–65.

the term. It is often said that by the 1930s eugenics was a pseudo-science already contradicted by modern genetic discoveries and discredited for political reasons, not the least of them being the emergence of extreme racist eugenics in Nazi Germany in 1933. What, then, are we to make of the fact that in Latin America eugenic activity intensified in the period?[63] The 1930s were, after all, as turbulent a period for Latin America as they were for Europe. Many countries experienced authoritarian, antidemocratic, even semifascist governments. I have already mentioned the right-wing military coup that removed Argentina's democratically elected government in 1930. The corporatist dictatorship that resulted was short-lived, but under the following conservative regimes of the 1930s, antidemocratic, extreme nationalist, and anti-Semitic ideologies flourished.[64] Brazil in the late 1930s saw the termination of all political parties, the suspension of democratic politics, and the development of a dictatorship with semifascist overtones in Getulio Vargas's "New State" (Estado Novo), a regime that lasted until the end of World War II. Of the three countries discussed here, only Mexico remained ideologically and publicly committed to progressive goals. Yet Mexico's nationalism, state-building, and antiforeign sentiment linked the country to other, ideologically very different nations of the region. Is the resurgence of eugenics in the 1930s, then, to be understood as a product of an authoritarian moment in Latin America, perhaps influenced by the development of fascist eugenics in Germany? Or should a different interpretation be put on eugenics in Latin America? What, in short, *was* Latin American eugenics? The next three chapters examine in some detail its preventive, sexual, and racial aspects.

63. Some historians have commented on the surprising resurgence of eugenics in the 1930s in "mainline" eugenic countries. On Britain, see G. R. Searle, "Eugenics and Politics in the 1930s," *Annals of Science* 36 (1979): 159–69.

64. David Rock, *Argentina, 1516–1982: From Spanish Colonization to the Falklands War* (Berkeley: University of California Press, 1985), p. 214.

3

Racial Poisons and the Politics of Heredity in Latin America in the 1920s

Science derives its political weight in the modern world from its conceptual claim to be a neutral, empirical, secular, and uniquely authoritative (because uniquely objective) form of knowledge.[1] Social conclusions or policies based on science often acquire, therefore, special legitimacy, precisely because of the assertion that they are natural extensions of science itself, derived in logical fashion from knowledge in a way other social ideas are not. Eugenists appealed implicitly to this kind of cognitive authority when they investigated social life and proposed social policies in the name of the science of heredity.

Yet, as historians, we are aware that neither theories of science nor their associated social conclusions are simple outcomes of neutral investigations. Both are, rather, bound up in mutually reinforcing systems of interpretation. Theories of nature are never merely discovered but are socially articulated; in turn, social conclusions derived from theories of nature are products of active interpretation, institution building, and the harnessing of political and cultural resources to give science certain meanings and to represent certain in-

1. For a good analysis, see Jack Morrell and Arnold Thackray, *Gentlemen of Science: Early Years of the British Association for the Advancement of Science* (Oxford: Clarendon Press, 1981), especially chap. 5.

terests.[2] In this chapter I analyze what mix of factors—political, cultural, and scientific—made some theories of heredity seem politically more compelling than others to the Latin American groups that called themselves eugenists. The kinds of social problems they highlighted as an outcome of their understanding of heredity, as well as the policies they viewed as correctives in the 1920s, must be seen in the wider context of the way supposedly objective knowledge of nature creates social meaning at a particular conjuncture in history.

The New Lamarckism in Latin America

A point of entry into Latin American eugenics is the remark by a British editor, K. E. Trounson, in 1931 on some Brazilian eugenic material sent to the British *Eugenics Review*. Trounson reported to his readers that "apparently the Brazilians interpret the word [eugenics] less strictly than we do, and make it cover a good deal of what we should call hygiene and elementary sexuology [sic], and no very clear distinction is drawn between congenital conditions due to prenatal injury and diseases which are strictly genetic." He added that, indeed, "genetics and natural and social selection are rather neglected; the outlook is more sociological than biological."[3]

Seen through British eyes, Brazilian eugenics may have seemed an example of misunderstanding or sloppy scientific thinking. From the Brazilian perspective, however, Trounson missed the underlying rationale of Brazilian eugenics. Brazilian eugenics in fact exemplified an important variant of the worldwide movement, one pervasive throughout Latin America but rarely included in accounts of eugenics. This variant was fundamentally non-Mendelian in outlook,

2. Morrell and Thackray, ibid., provide a brilliant example of the formation of modern scientific epistemology and ideology in the particular setting of Britain in the mid-nineteenth century; in Britain, science was conceptualized not only as abstract, neutral, empirical, etc., but as a "gentleman's" pursuit (hence the title of their book). One could extend the analysis to show how gender and race, in addition to class, were implicated in the formation of modern notions of science; science was, that is, seen as the learned and objective work of mainly European males who were capable of the high degree of rationality and abstraction science demanded. On this latter point see Nancy Leys Stepan and Sander L. Gilman, "Appropriating the Idioms of Science: Some Strategies of Resistance to Biological Determinism," in *The Bounds of Race: Perspectives on Hegemony and Resistance*, ed. Dominick LaCapra (Ithaca: Cornell University Press, 1991), pp. 72–103.

3. K. E. Trounson, "The Literature Reviewed," *Eugenics Review* 13 (1931): 236.

one that was both a result of, and productive of, particular social values. The failure to identify this variant is largely due to the fact that in the countries where eugenics has been most studied, Mendelism provided the apparently necessary foundations for a program of eugenics. In Britain, for instance, eugenics was very closely associated with Weismann's and Mendel's theories, which gave apparent precision and certainty to claims about the significance and meaning of heredity. The new genetics caused eugenists to turn from social reforms to biological ones, on the understanding that social reforms were limited in their effects to a single generation. With the rejection of Lamarckian notions of the inheritance of acquired characters there often came a sharp distinction between "nature" (heredity) and "nurture." The eugenists emphasized control over breeding, rather than reform of the social environment, as the natural conclusion to be derived from the new science of heredity. As the German eugenist Wilhelm Schallmayer put it, "Eugenics is the hygiene of the genotype while personal hygiene is that of the phenotype."[4]

Many of the doctors and reformers who were drawn into eugenics in Latin America were not readily persuaded of the correctness of the Weismannian-Mendelian point of view, however. This was less a matter of their being "out" of the mainstream of genetics than of their being "in" an alternative stream or tradition of Lamarckian hereditarian thought. The centrality of Mendelism to our modern genetics has made it easy to overlook the continued vitality of non-Mendelian ideas in medicine and science until well into the 1940s. The story of the persistence of neo-Lamarckian heredity is one that has not been told until recently, discredited as it is by its association with the excessive partisanship of Soviet scientists in the 1940s. Lysenkoism is often held up as the paradigmatic example of the distortions in science caused by crass political ideology. Because Trofim Denisovich Lysenko embraced Lamarckism for apparently political reasons and persecuted Mendelians and deformed Soviet genetics in the process, it has been easy to think of all Lamarckians of the twentieth century as left-wing ideologues and bad scientists to boot, because biology shows Lamarckian inheritance does not in fact occur.[5] Since the Soviet Lamarckians also attacked eugenics as a

4. Quoted in Jorge A. Frías, *El matrimonio, sus impedimientos y nulidades (derechos comparados)* (Córdoba, Argentina: Ateneo, 1941), p. 149.
5. On Lysenko's impact on Soviet genetics, see David Joravsky, *The Lysenko*

"bourgeois" science riddled with metaphysical, class, and racial biases, a eugenics movement based on Lamarckian heredity has until recently been treated almost as a contradiction in terms.

Yet the history of science shows us that competing paradigms in science are normal, that rarely does one scientific theory dominate all others in the field, and that no science escapes the political values of the society in which it is produced.[6] It also shows that the eventual consensus that may build up around one theory at the expense of other contenders is also rarely a simple matter concerning the superior logic or evidential basis of its claims, but a complicated social process involving networks of people, the construction of institutions, the making of political strategies, and the carrying out of a series of informal negotiations about meaning.[7] Because the history of science tends to get written from our present science backward—or as the historian Jan Sapp says, by the "victors"—those moments when values and theories are in conflict are underanalyzed.[8] This has been especially true in the history of genetics, where the sheer success of Mendelism, especially in its modern molecular biological form, has made it easy to forget those periods and places where other approaches to human heredity existed, as well as

---

Affair (Chicago: University of Chicago Press, 1970). Because Lysenko has been used as the exemplary case study of ideology producing bad science, it has been easy to propose that good science is nonideological or escapes the value system of the larger surroundings in which science is practiced. A middle way between these two extremes, whereby we can imagine that science is both reflective of social values in some mediated way and yet achieves an acceptable degree of objectivity, seems to be required.

6. See Ernst Mayr, *The Growth of Biological Thought: Diversity, Evolution, and Inheritance* (Cambridge, Mass.: Harvard University Press, 1982), p. 842; see also Larry Laudan, *Progress and Its Problems: Toward a Theory of Scientific Growth* (Berkeley: University of California Press, 1977), p. 75.

7. This view of science reflects many currents in the history and sociology of science. The key figure is Thomas S. Kuhn, who in *The Structure of Scientific Revolutions* (Chicago: University of Chicago Press, 1962) decisively changed our view of science by suggesting that scientific knowledge did not change merely because of the superior "truthfulness" or logic of succeeding theories or "paradigms." Since Kuhn, many others have contributed to the discussion.

8. Jan Sapp, "The Struggle for Authority in the Field of Heredity, 1900–1932: New Perspectives on the Rise of Genetics," *Journal of the History of Biology* 16 (Fall 1983): 311–42; see also his book *Beyond the Gene: Cytoplasmic Inheritance and the Struggle for Authority in Genetics* (New York: Oxford University Press, 1987).

the processes by which these interpretations were eventually marginalized in political and scientific circles.[9]

New historical work is increasingly revealing to us that the history of science is not linear but full of diverging and converging
lines, and struggles over interpretation and meaning; it also shows
that the story of how different sciences are given saliency in a particular setting is a matter of political values as well as institutional
power. The question addressed here is what gave Lamarckian theories of heredity and eugenics their political and cultural valency in
Latin America.[10]

A Neo-Lamarckian Medical Tradition

Of Lamarckism it has been said that "perhaps no biological hy-
pothesis has been tested so thoroughly and abandoned with such
reluctance."[11] Why was this so? What explains the deep appeal of a
theory of inheritance which scientists today believe to be false? Until
1859, the year Charles Darwin published *The Origin of Species*, Jean
Baptiste Pierre Antoine de Monet, the chevalier de Lamarck, was
remembered as a French biologist who fifty years earlier had produced the first systematic, scientific theory of "transformism," a
radical theory of evolution of successive forms of species. In
Lamarck's vast and to many mid-nineteenth-century minds unat-
tractively speculative scheme, the "inheritance of acquired characters" with which Lamarck's name is now irrevocably associated provided the mechanism by which changes induced in a living
organism from the outside could be handed on to future genera-

9. In one of the more radically revisionist histories of modern genetics, Sapp
argues that the rapid institutionalization of Mendelian genetics in the United States
must be understood not as merely a natural result of the correctness of Mendelian
science but as a social result of the Mendelians' deliberate exclusion of alternative
viewpoints, an exclusion achieved by the control of scientific institutions and the
political and economic resources that went into them. He proposes that we think of
the Mendelians as involved in a "struggle for authority" in a new arena of science,
carving out space for new scientific interpretations of nature. See Sapp, *Beyond the
Gene* [note 8], esp. chaps. 2 and 8.

10. See D. Buican, *Histoire de la génétique et de l'évolutionisme en France* (Paris:
Presses Universitaires de France, 1984).

11. Conway Zirkle, *Evolution, Marxian Biology, and the Social Scene* (Philadelphia:
University of Pennsylvania Press, 1959), p. 128.

tions, thereby causing transmutation. The classic example is of the giraffe, which stretched its neck up to reach its food and transformed itself over time into a long-necked species.[12]

After Darwin published *The Origin of Species*, Lamarckism enjoyed renewed popularity as an alternative explanation of evolution to Darwin's. Against Darwin's theory of random variation, struggle for survival and natural selection, a model of change that seemed to take all design out of the universe, Lamarckism counterposed an evolution driven by slow, purposeful adaptation to changes in the environment. It was an evolution that therefore seemed less brutal, less impersonal, and more humane than that proposed by the English naturalist. Previously regarded a marginal figure in French biology whose work had not been reissued since his death in 1829, Lamarck was now claimed as the real "father" of evolution. For decades after 1859, prominent thinkers in Great Britain, from Herbert Spencer to Samuel Butler and Bernard Shaw, as well as the majority of French scientists (who did not readily adopt Darwinian views for a variety of scientific, political, and nationalistic reasons) defended Lamarck's philosophy and the inheritance of acquired characters against the Darwinian outlook. In fields as diverse as anthropology, the social sciences, human evolution, psychiatry, and even the new psychoanalysis, Lamarckian ideas of heredity and evolution continued to play important interpretive roles.[13]

At the turn of the century, following first Weismann's work on the continuity of the germ plasm and then the rediscovery of Men-

12. On Lamarck's place in the history of evolutionary thought, see Richard W. Burkhardt, *The Spirit of the System: Lamarck and Evolutionary Biology* (Cambridge: Harvard University Press, 1977); for a brief account, see L. Jordanova, *Lamarck* (New York: Oxford University Press, 1984).

13. Jordanova, *Lamarck* [note 12], pp. 100–112. For an extensive general discussion of Lamarckism in biology in the late nineteenth century, see Peter J. Bowler, *The Eclipse of Darwin: Anti-Darwinism in the Decades around* 1900 (Baltimore: Johns Hopkins University Press, 1983). The American school of Lamarckian evolutionists, involving such biologists as Alpheus Hyatt, Alpheus S. Packard, and Edward Drinker Cope, is analyzed in James R. Moore, *The Post-Darwinian Controversies* (Cambridge: Cambridge University Press, 1979), pp. 141–52; see also Edward J. Pfeifer, "United States," in *The Comparative Reception of Darwinism*, ed. Thomas F. Glick (Chicago: University of Chicago Press, 1988), pp. 168–206. For the influence of Lamarckism on American anthropology and social sciences, see George W. Stocking, Jr., *Race, Culture, and Evolution: Essays in the History of Evolution* (London: Collier-Macmillan, 1968). For Freud's use of Lamarckian ideas, see his *Phylogenetic Fantasy* (Cambridge: Belknap Press of Harvard University Press, 1985).

del's laws of inheritance in 1900, Lamarckism became a subject of more active dispute in biological circles. Weismann was particularly important to the story of Lamarckism because he seemed to offer experimental proof that the inheritance of acquired characterists did not occur. Heredity was therefore "hard," not "soft" as traditionally believed. Lamarckians protested, as Peter Bowler notes, that the acquired characteristics they had in mind were not the brutal mutilations with which Weismann had experimented, but subtle, slow, internal, adaptive changes of the organism to the environment.[14] But Weismann's approach had the effect of forcing the Lamarckians to come to terms with the new findings of the Weismann-Mendelians and to try to give experimental precision to their own contrasting views of the laws of inheritance.

Lamarkism, at first a general, early-nineteenth-century theory of transformism, was itself transformed into a "neo"-Lamarckism.[15] After the rediscovery of Mendelian laws of inheritance in 1900, Lamarckism narrowed still further to mean a particular theory of how inheritance worked. The theory continued to be employed because it offered a reasonable alternative to the continued uncertainties in genetics and to what many biologists thought were the exaggerated claims of the Weismannites. Scepticism among biologists about strict Mendelism was not confined to any single country. According to a recent account of evolutionary biology in Germany, in 1912 "no one doubted the possibility of an induction of germ cells by external stimuli," meaning by "induction" the capacity of some agency outside the genetic material itself to alter the character of that material.[16] The experimentalist Paul Kammerer was one of the best-known of the neo-Lamarckians; he died by suicide in 1926 after the revelation that his experimental data in favor of the inheritance of acquired characteristics had apparently been faked. His death may have sealed the fate of neo-Lamarckism in the history books, but not in history.[17] In Britain, the biologists E. W. McBride and H. C.

14. Peter J. Bowler, *Evolution: The History of an Idea* (Berkeley: University of California Press, 1984), pp. 238–39.

15. The term was first used by the American biologist Alphonse Packard in 1885.

16. Bernhard Rensch, in *Dimensions of Darwinism: Themes and Counter-Themes in Twentieth Century Evolutionary Theory*, ed. Majorie G. Grene (Cambridge: Cambridge University Press, 1983), pp. 31–42.

17. For an entertaining, partisan, but not always accurate account of the Kammerer "affair," see Arthur Koestler, *The Midwife Toad* (New York: Vintage, 1973).

Cannon, as well as such medical doctors as Saleeby, continued to take the minority, neo-Lamarckian position well into the 1930s, in the face of the majority endorsement of the Mendelian point of view.

Their Lamarckism was a position with which many Latin American scientists and physicians agreed, but not because Latin Americans were, by nature or culture, unscientific or out of touch. Individual Latin American scientists often showed themselves to be suprisingly au courant with new developments in genetics. In Argentina, for example, Alfredo Binbarén gave an account of Galton's statistical law, the "coefficient of regression," in 1886, the very year it appeared in the *Proceedings* of the Royal Society.[18] Binbarén described the individual as a "mosaic of hereditary characters" that are independent of one another. He also concluded that "the Jews" showed heredity at work in their inheritance of an affinity for wealth; and he wrote of his country's need for "pure blood"— his remarks revealing to us how quickly the new genetics would be given a eugenic-racist slant. Angel Gallardo, another early student of Mendelism, in 1908 brought together in a short book a review of the latest developments in genetics—Galton's laws, the life and work of Mendel, Hugo De Vries's theory of mutation, the dispute between the Mendelians and biometricians in Britain, and Charles Davenport's conversion to Mendelism, the author referring yet again to the "triumph of the new concept of race and pure blood."[19] By 1917 the first university course in Mendelian genetics was being given by Miguel Hernández, a zoologist at the University of La Plata.[20] In Mexico, the zoologist and evolutionist Alfonso L. Herrera

18. A. Binbarén, "La ley de la herencia," *Anales del Instituto Agronómico-Veterinario de la Provincia de Buenos Aires* 1 (August 20, 1886): 17–19; (September 5): 37–39; (September 20): 59–60; (October 5): 84; (October 20): 103–4; and (November 5): 123–24.

19. Angel Gallardo, *Las investigaciones modernas sobre la herencia en biología* (Buenos Aires: Ciencia Médica, 1908). This book of fifty-eight pages has a twelve-page bibliography. Gallardo had reviewed developments in genetics for several years by the time this book appeared; his earliest book appeared in French as *Les mathématiques et la biologie* (Paris, 1901). For an evaluation, see Luis B. Mazoti and Juan H. Hunziker, "Los precursores iniciadores de la genética en la Argentina," in *Evolución de las ciencias en la República Argentina, 1923–1972*, 4 vols. (Buenos Aires: Sociedad Científica Argentina, 1976), 4:5–12.

20. Alberto Boerger, "La genética contemporánea del Rio de la Plata," *Ciencia e Investigación* 9 (1953): 435–45. A Spanish translation of Mendel's original paper appeared in Argentina in 1934; it was undertaken by the agronomist Arturo Burkart

made a very brief mention of Mendel's laws in his textbook *Ideas of Biology* (*Nociones de biología*), which he prepared for teaching purposes in 1904.[21] In Brazil, a medical thesis on neo-Lamarckism written in 1907 indicates that some of the younger medical students were already being introduced to the genetic debates current in Europe.[22] The first book on Mendelism per se and the new science of hybridization was published in 1917 by Carlos Teixeira Mendes, a professor at the Agricultural School of Piracicaba in the state of São Paulo.[23] The social significance of the competing theories of inheritance was also recognized; indeed, genetic theory was usually introduced together with eugenics.[24] In 1925 Gonçalo Moniz was one of the first in Brazil to introduce Mendelian ideas in a more popular way in Bahia, in a book defending consanguineous marriages.[25]

In Latin America, Mendelian genetics was taken up by agricultural and horticultural institutions located in the richer agricultural regions where animal and plant breeding were important. Elsewhere, though, Mendelism tended to be marginal until the late 1930s. The neo-Lamarckian inflections in heredity involved less matters of fact or logic than factors of culture and politics, which are

---

and was published in the *Revista Argentina de Agricultura* 1(1) (1934): 1–38. Burkart was a disciple of Curt Stern, with whom he worked in 1928 at the Kaiser Wilhelm Institute in Berlin, and was the first to work on the fruit fly, *Drosophila melanogaster*, in Argentina, beginning in 1931. The strongest tradition of Mendelism in the country was in plant genetics.

21. Alfonso L. Herrera, *Nociones de biología* (Mexico City: Secretario de Fomento, 1904), pp. 216–17. A footnote said that this portion was not obligatory for students. Enrique Beltrán, in "Cándido Bolívar Pieltain y los biólogos españoles en México," *Revista de la Sociedad Mexicana de Historia Natural* 27 (December 1976): 19–28, mentions an early work by Cosio, published in the *Gazeta Médica de México* 5 (1910): 40–45, on the inheritance of transmissible diseases, which Beltrán says demonstrated an adequate grasp of Mendelism as well as knowledge about the work of De Vries and Lucien Cuénot.

22. João Florentino Meira, *Neo-Lamarckismo* (Rio de Janeiro: Carvalhaes, 1907). This work was presented at the Rio Medical School; the thesis reviewed neo-Darwinian ideas (as expressed in George Romanes's *Darwin and After Darwin*, 3 vols. [London: Longmans, Green, 1892–1897]) as well as neo-Lamarckian ones, but it endorsed the neo-Lamarckian position.

23. Carlos Teixeira Mendes, *Melhoramento de variedades agrícolas* (Piracicaba: Livraria Americana, 1917). A medical thesis on Mendelism was written the next year; see Luiz Viana, "Em torno do Mendelismo" (Ph.D. diss., Nitheroi, 1918).

24. For example, Viana's doctoral thesis, "Em torno do Mendelismo" [note 23], contained a long section on eugenics.

25. Gonçalo Moniz, *A consanguinidade e o código civil brasileiro* (Bahia, 1925). A slightly later discussion of Mendel and eugenics was Pedro Monteleone's *Os cinco problemas da eugenia brasileira* (São Paulo: Irmãos Gibin, 1929), esp. pp. 21–25.

ineluctably part of science. One such factor was the integration of many Latin American doctors into a continental tradition of science which for a number of reasons was highly Lamarckian.[26] In France, especially, Lamarckism remained authoritative not just in the early part of the twentieth century, when many biologists were doubtful of Mendelism and when natural selection theory was at its nadir, but throughout the 1920s, 1930s, and well into the 1940s.

As the Mexican zoologist and historian of Mexican science Enrique Beltrán has commented, by tradition Latin Americans looked to France for their scientific ideas.[27] French was the second language of the educated elite, and many foreign works in science came to the region in French translation. French biology was therefore the natural cultural source of new biological-social ideas, a source reflected in the fact that the names invariably cited by the Latin Americans were French authorities—Adolphe Pinard, Frédéric Houssay, Louis Landouzy, Edmond Perrier, Emile Guyenot, Charles Richet, and Eugène Apert. Until the 1920s it was to France that Latin American students of science and medicine went if they could for their medical and biological training, and it was there that they aspired to be published and recognized.[28] As a result of these linguistic and cultural ties, biological ideas often came to Latin America from France, and deeply tinged with Lamarckian colors.[29] It is no accident, for instance, that Alfonso L. Herrera first published his work on evolutionary biology in French.[30] No accident, either, that though he was

26. See Bowler, *Eclipse of Darwin* [note 13], and Sapp, *Beyond the Gene* [note 8]. Some French biologists were exceptions to the neo-Lamarckian orientation, e.g., Cuénot. See Denis Buican, "Mendelism in France and the Work of Lucien Cuénot," *Scientia* 117 (1982): 129–36.

27. Beltrán, "Cándido Bolívar Pieltain" [note 21], p. 19.

28. In the physical sciences the situation was rather different; here Britain and Germany were more important reference points for Latin Americans. See Lewis Pyenson and M. Singli, "Physics on the Periphery: A World Survey, 1920–1929," *Scientometrics* 6 (1984): 279–306.

29. A late edition of the Mexican biologist I. Ochoterena's *Tratado elemental de biología* (Mexico City: Botas, 1950) still placed Lamarck with Darwin as the greatest innovator in biology. Another important source of Lamarckian ideas in Latin America was Ernst Haeckel's work, which had a large impact in the region; see Julio Orione, "Florentino Ameghino y la influencia de Lamarck en la paleontología argentina del siglo XIX," *Quipu: Revista Latinoamericana de Historia de las Ciencias y la Tecnología* 4 (1987): 447–71.

30. Alfonso L. Herrera, "La vie sur les hauts plateaux: Influence de la pression barométrique sur la constitution et le développement des êtres organisés; Traitement climatérique de la tuberculose" (Mexico City: El Escalante, 1899). Herrera's first

a declared Darwinist, Herrera took Lamarck as the founding figure of evolutionism and combined Darwinian struggle with the inheritance of acquired characteristics.[31]

Like the French biologists to whom they turned for scientific guidance, the Latin Americans had a variety of reasons, some explicit and some implicit, for preferring neo-Lamarckian views over strict Darwinian, Weismannian, and Mendelian ones. An examination of these reasons does much to explain the enduring appeal of the neo-Lamarckian approach to evolution and heredity in Latin America. Philosophically, Weismannism was unattractive to Latin American biologists because it implied to them a determinism that seemed to leave no place for individual will and action in the development of human society. Along with their French counterparts, they could not accept the absolute separation between soma and germ plasm demanded by Weismannians and strict Mendelians. Politically, neo-Lamarckism also often came tinged with an optimistic expectation that reforms of the social milieu would result in permanent improvement, an idea in keeping with the environmentalist-sanitary tradition that had become fashionable in the area. The leader of Mexican eugenics, Dr. Alfredo Saavedra, for instance, called the idea of the germ plasm a fantasy and vowed to combat it, citing the biologist Paul Kammerer, among the Europeans, and Fernando Ocaranza in Mexico as having dedicated themselves to countering Weismann's evil influence on biology.[32] The biologist I. Ochoterena, Saavedra's contemporary, expressed the same skepticism, commenting that "if the body undergoes changes it affects all parts, including the reproductive cells. This gives reality to the ideal of Lamarck."[33] The engineer and eugenist Adalberto García de Mendoza criticized both Weismannism *and* dialectical materialism— Weismannism because it insisted that the germ plasm was unaltered by the environment and dialectic materialism because it ignored the

---

textbook was also published in Mexico in French; see A. L. Herrera, *Receuil des lois de la biologie générale* (Mexico City: Secretaria de Fomento, 1897).

31. See Alfonso L. Herrera's French version of his early biology textbook, *Notions générales de biologie* (Berlin: W. Junk, 1906), p. 133, where Herrera excluded mutilations (e.g., amputations, circumcision) as modifications that are inherited, but included acquired modifications that affected the entire organism, such as malaria, tuberculosis, vices, perturbations of nutrition, and alcohol.

32. Alfredo Saavedra, "Lo 'eugénico' anunciado por primera vez en México," *Acción Médica* 199 (September 1956): 16–17.

33. Ochoterena, *Tratado elemental de biología* [note 29], p. 256.

reality of "transcendental values" that existed in the individual and the human collectivity.[34]

Such philosophical-political dislike of strict Weismannism was often reinforced by the objections of the religiously inclined to what was viewed as the rank materialism of the Darwinian point of view; since, according to Lamarckism, evolution was the result not of blind material forces but of changes brought about by will and choice, Lamarckism was seen as more in keeping with traditional ideas of morality and was embraced for this reason. It allowed, as the British Saleeby put it, "a recognition of a positive factor, which is not mechanical but psychical."[35] A Lamarckian style of evolution seemed a gentler, more harmonious and humane way of perfecting nature than one based on Darwin's brutish struggle. To a neo-Lamarckian, natural selection might result in a weeding out of the unfit variations, but the inheritance of acquired characters was responsible for the origin of the fittest. Politically, neo-Lamarckian ideas justified the belief that human effort had meaning, that improvements acquired in an individual's lifetime could be handed on genetically, that progress could occur.

And last, as a theory of heredity per se, Lamarckism provided an apparent solution to the continued uncertainties surrounding the mechanism of inheritance.[36] Doubt was particularly strong in Latin American medical circles, where the French influence was especially powerful. In Brazil, for instance, the National Academy of Medicine and the Faculty of Medicine in Rio de Janeiro were both modeled on the French examples. In 1908 a Peruvian physician went so far as to call the French influence in medicine "absolute," saying that "texts from this country [France] are practically the only ones the students study."[37] The continued reliance on scientifically refined but La-

34. Adalberto García de Mendoza, "La eugenesia frente a los problemas sociales contemporáneas," *Boletín de La Sociedad Eugénica Mexicana* 10 (October 20, 1932): 4.

35. Caleb W. Saleeby, as quoted in Greta Jones, *Social Darwinism and English Thought: The Interaction of Biological and Social Theory* (Sussex: Harvester, 1980), p. 94. See Bowler's reference in *Evolution* [note 14], p. 244, to the "inner theology" contained in Lamarckism, based on the feeling that "living things are in charge of their own evolution; they *choose* their response to each environmental challenge and thus direct their own evolution."

36. On Darwin's own "Lamarckism," see Bowler, *Evolution* [note 14], pp. 161, 178.

37. David Matto, *La enseñanza médica en el Perú* (Lima: El Lucero, 1908), p. 35. I have Marcos Cueto to thank for this reference.

marckian ideas by French, and by extension Latin American, physicians reflected not ignorance but an alternative tradition of political, scientific and philosophical concerns as well as the seemingly intractable problems of human pathology. Charles Rosenberg has pointed out that Lamarckism provided a flexible model of disease etiology that underscored the physician's own agency.[38] Mendelism did not seem to provide such interpretive and medical flexibility and for this reason did not immediately displace Lamarckism. Take, for example, the impact of parental health and disease on reproduction. Did the child of ill parents not suffer in fitness, and was not this unfitness transmitted by an acquired heredity?[39] It had long been known, for instance, that children of syphilitic parents could suffer from infantile syphilis, a condition usually attributed to the inheritance of acquired characters, the result of defective sperm or ovum. Such a notion had already been made the basis for caution in marriage choices in the late nineteenth century; by the early twentieth century, as the advent of Mendelism changed the context of genetic debate, infantile syphilis was often used as an argument for the reality of Lamarckian inheritance.[40] The same could be said of alcoholism. Could not a hereditary alcoholic condition be created in a child by the parents' heavy drinking, and would not this condition, once established in the hereditary makeup of the child, be transmitted thereafter to the next generation, in the form of either alcoholism itself or other weaknesses and pathologies? Could not even infectious diseases, caused by known microorganisms, also at times cause defects in a child which were not what we would call "congenital," and confined to the individual offspring, but permanent, marking the hereditary material over several generations?

Even in circles where Mendelism represented the dominant view, doctors continued to show considerable uncertainty about how far to push the new Weismanism-Mendelism at the expense of the older, more traditional versions of inheritance. At the Second International Congress of Eugenics, held in New York in 1921 under the aegis of the aggressively "Mendelian" U.S. eugenists, a physician,

38. Charles E. Rosenberg, *No Other Gods: On Science and American Social Thought* (Baltimore: Johns Hopkins University Press, 1976), chap. 1.

39. Elizabeth Lomax, "Infantile Syphilis as an Example of Nineteenth Century Belief in the Inheritance of Acquired Characteristics," *Journal of the History of Medicine* 34 (January 1979): 23–39.

40. Ibid.

William S. Sadler, reported on the results of a questionnaire he had sent to two hundred geneticists, eugenists, biologists, and neurologists asking what they believed about the ability of external poisons to cause permanent alterations in the germ plasm; he showed that 60 percent believed such poisons could have effects that persisted through successive generations. Sadler concluded that the puzzling exceptions to Mendelism could not be overlooked. At the same congress a British authority on mental deficiency, Dr. Arthur F. Tredgold, said he had similar doubts about strict Mendelism; many facts inclined him to Lamarckian views.[41]

From "Homiculture" to Eugenics

Neo-Lamarckian ideas formed the context in which long-standing preoccupations with progress, health, and nationality converged in the new eugenics institutions of Latin America, in a social and scientific process that lasted several years. By tracing this process, we can capture the scientific and political circumstances by which the distinctive form of Latin American eugenics developed. The history of the word "homiculture" provides one way into that process. The word was introduced into medical debate in Latin America in 1911 by two Cuban physicians, Eusebio Hernández and Domingo F. Ramos, as a way of conceptualizing the new medical understanding of the role of heredity in human society.[42] "Homiculture" was connected to, and indeed was a play on, another word popular in medical circles at the time, "puericulture"; and the book's dedication to the well-known French obstetrician and puericulturist Adolphe Pinard revealed clearly the Cubans' debt to French medicine and the

41. William S. Sadler, "Endocrines, Defective Germ-Plasm, and Hereditary Defectiveness," in *Eugenics, Genetics, and the Family* (New York: Williams and Wilkins, 1923), pp. 341–50; Tredgold, p. 369; M. T. Nisot, in the review of eugenics in 1927, *La question eugénique dans divers pays* (Brussels: Faille, 1927), p. 17, stated that at this congress it was established scientifically that the deterioration of germ plasm was indeed caused by alcohol, toxins, and radioactivity.

42. Eusebio Hernández and Domingo F. Ramos, *Homicultura* (Havana: Secretaria de Sanidad y Beneficencia, 1911). This word, for which Ramos always claimed originality, was actually a modification of "hominiculture," which the French physician Landouzy used to refer to the battle against the three "poisons" of alcohol, syphilis, and tuberculosis.

distinctive roots of French and Latin American eugenics. From homiculture would emerge the new eugenics.[43]

Pinard was the professor of clinical obstetrics at the School of
Medicine and headed the Baudelocque Clinic in Paris (founded in
1890 and named after an earlier French authority on obstetrics). He
was, wrote the Cubans, the creator of the science of "puericulture."[44]
Actually, puericulture, or the scientific cultivation of the child, did
not originate with Pinard (the term had been introduced as early as.
1865), but Pinard had given it new vigor in the mid-1890s as a way
of dealing with what many doctors in France perceived were the
manifold problems of low rates of reproduction and the continued
high rates of infant and maternal mortality and morbidity.[45] Pronatalism was already a prominent theme in France, and the physicians joined in a national debate about the causes of the nation's low
fertility rate, a debate that intensified after the defeat of France in the
Franco-Prussian War and as statistical studies showed that France
apparently had the lowest fertility rate in Europe.[46] Many doctors
concluded that France's population growth was too low to permit
the French to compete economically and militarily with the Germans. There was a growing belief that women's work outside the
home and the continued high incidence of disease among the working class were creating a veritable crisis of "depopulation" which
could best be tackled by medical policies. Pronatalism and medicine
thus became linked together in puericulture. French obstetricians,
following Pinard's lead, thought of mothers and children as forming
a kind of reproductive, collective political economy whose health
was vital to the nation. As Jane Ellen Crisler says, the word "puericulture" was in fact a kind of human analogue to "agriculture."[47]

Pinard defined puericulture as the investigation of knowledge re-

43. The term remained part of Latin American eugenic discourse, being used, for
example, in the Pan American conferences on eugenics and homiculture in 1927 and
1934.

44. Hernández and Ramos, *Homicultura* [note 42].

45. William Schneider, "Toward the Improvement of the Human Race: The History of Eugenics in France," *Journal of Modern History* 54 (June 1982): 268–91.

46. Karen Offen, "Depopulation, Nationalism, and Feminism in Fin-de-Siècle
France," *American Historical Review* 89 (1984): 648–76.

47. Jane Ellen Crisler, "'Saving the Seed': The Scientific Preservation of Children
in France during the Third Republic" (Ph.D. diss., University of Wisconsin–Mad-
ison, 1984), p. 76.

lating to reproduction and the conservation and improvement of the human species. Based on the nineteenth-century notion that acquired characters could become hereditary, Pinard's revival of puericulture focused physicians' attention on the importance of maternal and child care for the future of the nation; Pinard emphasized especially the significance of the very moment of conception, when factors in the parents' environment were believed to be especially threatening to the health of offspring. Fatigue, "poisons" such as nicotine and alcohol, and a poor diet, had negative effects on the condition of the germinal materials, he argued, risking the mother's own health at childbirth as well as the health of the child. The task of the obstetrician and the pediatrician was to reduce all the adverse factors threatening health in reproduction, through sexual education, aid to families, and new obstetric techniques. Puericulture made the mother-child unit the special site of medical attention, and obstetrics, gynecology, and pediatrics the paramount medical specialities. Children especially were thought of as biological-political resources of the nation, and the state was regarded as having an obligation to regulate their health. Rooted as puericulture was in a profoundly traditional view of the woman's role in the family and reproduction, the puericulturists focused on the need to keep women *in* reproduction, healthily rearing their children according to modern medical principles for the good of the country.

By the early twentieth century, the word "puericulture" had become common in French and Latin American medical circles. Physicians' attraction to puericulture followed from the dependence of Latin American medicine on French leads. In addition, the Latin American countries shared with France several political characteristics that gave support to the notion of puericulture: an emphasis on agriculture and the resonance of agricultural metaphors of cultivation, a pronatalism based on high maternal and infant mortality rates and the consequent worry about inadequate population growth, and an essentially conservative, profamily outlook.

Hernández had gone to Paris from Havana in 1889 to study directly under Pinard. Hernández's career, like the careers of so many Cuban physicians of his generation, was interrupted by the Cuban war of independence from Spain, a war in which Hernández participated for three years. The war eventually ended when the United States entered the war against Spain and formally occupied Havana in January 1899; thereafter the United States played an important and not always welcome role in overseeing the health of the new republic.[48] Before this date, Hernández had already returned to France for further work with Pinard and the new puericulture. On his return to Cuba he published a book on the topic of homiculture; it carried a preface by the secretary of health, who hoped thereby to persuade the president of Cuba to begin a practical health campaign.

Hernández and Ramos proposed the word "homiculture" as a substitute for "puericulture." Homiculture, as the Cubans saw it, was larger than puericulture, since "homiculture" referred to the scientific cultivation of the entire individual, from before birth to adulthood, and not just the child. Homiculture was schematically divided into several parts: "patrimatriculture" (the culture of the parents), "matrifeticulture" (the care of the pregnant mother and the fetus together), puericulture itself, "progonoculture" (care of the gonads), and "post-genitoculture" (care of the individual after birth). This schema indicated, Ramos thought, the proper place of puericulture within the more spacious field of homiculture. The clumsy, overelaborate, and inconsistent terminology, derived from Pinard with modifications, found few adherents in Latin America, though it was kept in the title of the Pan American meetings of eugenics which Ramos later organized. The term "homiculture" did, however, have the advantage of drawing attention to the fact that whereas "puericulture" referred to the care of the *child* before and after birth, "homiculture" included the care of the future parents from birth to adulthood and the health of their "gonads" (gonoculture) and of the fetus from the moment of conception. In short, the terms made clear that homiculture encompassed all of the problems of heredity surrounding human reproduction.

Homiculture represented, as it were, one stage on the road from the puericulture of the late nineteenth century to the more radical and innovative neo-Lamarckian eugenics of the early twentieth, and reflected the growing hereditarianism of medical thought in the period. In 1899 Pinard had already begun to redefine his notion of puericulture as "puericulture before birth," thereby giving an emphasis to the special problem of parental influences on the hereditary

48. On these events, especially in relation to health, see Nancy Stepan, "The Interplay between Socio-Economic Factors and Medical Science: Yellow Fever Research, Cuba, and the United States," *Social Studies of Science* 8 (1978): 397–423.

condition of the offspring.[49] The full transformation of puericulture into a neo-Lamarckian eugenics in France occurred when a group of French physicians founded the French Eugenics Society in Paris.

This society was a direct outcome of French participation in the First International Eugenics Congress, held in London in July 1912. There the French delegation of puericulturists, alienists, social scientists and biologists came into contact with British and other "Anglo-Saxon" eugenists. Though Pinard did not attend in person, owing to illness, he prepared a paper on the aspect of puericulture most closely connected to heredity—that is, puericulture before birth. Six months after the delegates returned to France, they formed their own eugenics organization.[50]

The French historian of medicine Jacques Léonard has commented that what was remarkable about the French Eugenics Society was how untouched it was by the new Mendelian genetics, and at least initially, by the maximalist or extreme social ideas of many of the Anglo-Saxon eugenists—that it remained faithful to its neo-Lamarckian, puericultural roots.[51] Léonard goes so far as to call its initial program "pure hygienism," its goal the prevention of the environment from being a source of hereditary degradation in humans and the sanitization and civilization of the reproductive instinct. Léonard missed the special gender implications of the new eugenics (implications explored in more detail in Chapter 4). But he is right to point out that Pinard's initial aim was not so much to stop the so-called unfit from breeding as to stimulate the growth of a fit population and to educate the largest number of people possible about the necessity of ensuring that procreation take place in healthy conditions. It was, in many respects, an original form of eugenics, and it had considerable resonance in Latin America, where its themes of

49. See Schneider, "Toward the Improvement of the Human Race" [note 45].

50. Adolphe Pinard, "Considerations générales sur 'La Puericulture avant la Procréation,'" in *Problems in Eugenics* (London: Eugenics Education Society, 1912), pp. 457–59.

51. See Jacques Léonard, "Le Premier Congrès International d'Eugénique (Londres, 1912) et ses consequences françaises," *Histoires des Sciences Médicales* 17 (1983): 141–46; and his "Eugénisme et Darwinisme: Espoirs et perplexités chez des médécins français du XIXe siècle et du début du XXe siècle," in *De Darwin au Darwinisme: Science et idéologie*, ed. Y. Conry (Paris: Vrin, 1983), pp. 187–207. For a full analysis of the French eugenics movement see William H. Schneider, *Quality and Quantity: The Quest for Biological Regeneration in Twentieth-Century France* (New York: Cambridge University Press, 1990).

neo-Lamarckian inheritance and "puericulture before birth" were re-iterated in all the main eugenics organizations.

In following Pinard into eugenics, many Latin American doctors saw their ideas as extending principles of public health into the special sphere of heredity in reproduction. Eschewing a hard-and-fast distinction between heredity and the environment, they paid considerable attention to the milieu in which reproduction occurred, because it was seen as a source of reproductive "poisons" that could have disastrous consequences for future generations. Eugenics thus became linked to obstetrics, population policies, and infant welfare, and made common cause with campaigns against alcoholism, tuberculosis, and venereal disease. The appeal of the new "puericulture before birth" cut across political lines. Everyone, it seemed, could agree that human reproduction was not only sacred but valuable to the state, that children needed protection, and that doctors had an obligation to sanitize and moralize the sexual sphere in order to make the nation healthy and strong. In revolutionary Mexico, for instance, the first classes on eugenics were given in 1919 by the holder of the newly created chair of puericulture, and the association of eugenics with puericulture continued in the two national conferences on the child held in 1921 and 1923, at which eugenics was given a highly controversial hearing.[52] When the Mexican Eugenics Society for the Improvement of Race finally came into being in 1931, it did so as a direct offshoot of the earlier Mexican Society of Puericulture (founded in 1929), in which a section of eugenics had been created. The name "puericulture" eventually disappeared in the eugenics society, but the themes of puericulture—the need to instruct potential parents on the hereditary risks of reproduction, the problem of protecting the health of the mother and child, the "right" of the child to be hereditarily "wellborn," the dangers of alcohol and other toxins on the fetus—were pursued under the banner of eugenics. In the quite differently organized Association of Biotypology, Eugenics, and Social Medicine in Buenos Aires— which, as we have seen, was founded in a period of conservative reaction—puericulture and heredity were similarly brought together in powerful combination, the name of the association capturing well the nexus of ideas in the Latin style.[53]

52. Saavedra, "Lo 'eugénico' anunciado por primera vez en México" [note 32].
53. This subject is discussed further in Chapter 4.

Earlier, in Brazil, the new São Paulo Eugenics Society, organized in 1918, had taken the French Eugenics Society as a direct model, the French statutes being reproduced word for word in the charter of the society. Renato Kehl commented much later that before 1918 Brazilian doctors had been ignorant of eugenics because the chief works were written in German and English.[54]

This neo-Lamarckian, puericulturist, and sanitation orientation influenced even eugenists who had considerable contact with Anglo-Saxon ideas about heredity and eugenics. In 1912 the Argentine doctor Victor Delfino gave a careful account in *La Semana Médica* (Medical Week), the journal he edited, of scientific and eugenic topics discussed at the meetings of the First International Congress of Eugenics in London. He was particularly clear about the controversies over biometrics and Mendelism.[55] Yet in the short-lived Argentine Eugenics Society he founded in 1918 with the help of the professor of puericulture at the Faculty of Medicine, Ubaldo Fernández, and Gregorio Aráoz Alfaro, professor of obstetrics, the neo-Lamarckian style of eugenics predominated, with its emphasis on puericulture and on the need to prevent "poisons" in the environment from damaging reproduction and heredity.[56] Delfino himself unconsciously grafted the language of Galton and Mendelism onto the older tradition of puericulture and neo-Lamarckism. Before World War I and after, even as his involvement with U.S. eugenists widened (he served as one of the vice presidents of the Second International Eugenics Congress in New York), his own writings were devoted to the dangers presented to the health of the human species by such toxins as tobacco.[57]

The same mix of languages and styles characterized the Argentine League of Social Prophylaxis, which replaced the small and short-lived Argentine Eugenics Society as the chief center of eugenics in the mid-1920s. The founder and president, the doctor Alfredo Fer-

54. The statutes are given in the *Annães de eugenía* (São Paulo: Revista do Brasil, 1919), preface. Kehl's remarks were made in his book *Eugenía e medicina social (problemas da vida)* (Rio de Janeiro: Francisco Alves, 1923), p. vi.

55. Victor Delfino, "La eugenía o eugénica. Una nueva ciencia. El Congreso de Londres," *Semana Médica* (December 1912): 1174–76; and "Consecuencias de la ley de Mendel. Interpretación de Herder. Terminología de Bates. Biometrías y Mendelianos. La pangénesis de Darwin," *Semana Médica* (July 1912): 175–77.

56. See Victor Delfino, "La eugénica en los Estados Unidos," *Semana Médica* (October 1919): 403–4. See Chapter 4 for further discussion.

57. See Victor Delfino, "El tabaco y el sistema nervioso," *Archivos Brasileiros de Medicina* 5 (1915): 291–306.

nández Verano, said he derived the transcendent importance of eugenics from Pinard; of all the terms canvassed for eugenics—"eugenics" itself, "stirpiculture," "hominiculture," "puericulture before conception"—Verano said he preferred the latter. Verano's understanding of the problem of eugenics, like Pinard's and Delfino's, revolved around the effect that chronic intoxicants, infectious diseases, and other factors could have in causing morbid heredity.[58]

The neo-Lamarckian basis of the Latin American eugenists was often hidden, even from themselves, by their constant reference to Galton as the "father" of eugenics and by the absence of any direct mention of Lamarck. The Brazilian Kehl, for example, referred to neo-Lamarckian and Mendelian genetics as though they were variations of the same science of heredity.[59] The eclectic style of much of the eugenic writings and the catholic use of sources—as when Galton's ancestral law was presented in conjunction with Mendel's without acknowledgment that the latter in fact contradicted the former—indicates that very few physicians saw any incompatability between neo-Lamarckian and other kinds of inheritance.[60] Such reconciliation of the languages of genetics was hardly peculiar to Latin American doctors. Bowler shows that the rediscovery of Mendel forced the neo-Lamarckians in the United States and Europe to delimit rather than abandon the idea of inheritance of acquired characteristics.[61] Very often, the Lamarckians accepted Mendelian laws of inheritance while leaving a space nonetheless for the idea that somehow an influence from the environment could permanently alter the germ plasm.[62] The language of the two kinds of inheritance merged, allowing eugenists to associate themselves with Mendelism without giving up their deep-seated belief that at least some acquired characteristics were inherited.

The neo-Lamarckian orientation of eugenics was seen very clearly

58. Alfredo Fernández Verano, *Las doctrinas eugénicas (ensayo de sistematización)* (Buenos Aires: Liga Argentina de Profilaxis Social, 1929), esp. pp. 6–10 and 12–13.

59. Renato Kehl, *Lições de eugenía* (Rio de Janeiro: Brasil, 1935), pp. 78–99.

60. Ibid., p. 107. On the inability of many eugenists to recognize the contradiction, see Garland Allan, "From Eugenics to Population Control: The Work of Raymond Pearl," *Science for the People* 12 (July/August 1980): 22–28.

61. Bowler, *Eclipse of Darwin* [note 13], pp. 75–76.

62. Joaquim José de Andrade Filho, in his book *Da genohygia no Brasil* (Rio de Janeiro: Jornal do Commercio, 1924), endorsed Mendelism but qualified his endorsement in typical fashion by remarking that "one cannot separate the organism from the environment" (p. 37); he also commented that Galton was erected on the pedestal of Lamarck.

in the Latin American physicians' attachment to Auguste Forel's theory of "blastophthoria," which was used to explain how alcohol, venereal diseases, and tuberculosis could cause actual hereditary decay. By the early twentieth century, blastophthoria had come to refer to a lesion of the germ plasm, or, as a student of eugenics and matrimony put it, a "supplanting of hereditary normality, so that illness, toxins, and certain diseases could change the hereditary determinants, causing defects in the offspring."[63] Blastophthoria was often differentiated from ordinary (Mendelian) heredity, which was viewed as acting only to conserve ancestral traits; blastophthoric factors outside the germ plasm were believed actually to alter hereditary traits, stamping their new character on their descendants. It was a concept well suited to merge with the language of Mendelism, while keeping a place for social and moral action in heredity.

By the second decade of the twentieth century, the range of accepted blastophthoric influences had narrowed. No longer did Latin American doctors pretend that gross mutilations or most infectious diseases acquired in an individual's lifetime were transmitted by heredity to the next generation. It was assumed that only the constant repetition of certain kinds of deleterious influences would subtly alter the germ plasm and cause it to deteriorate. Alcohol, venereal diseases, tuberculosis, and toxins such as lead and tobacco were the factors most usually cited as blastophthoric in their effects. On the latter point there was almost universal agreement—that alcoholism, for example, was not just a sign of a preexisting hereditary degeneracy but a potential cause of a new hereditary predisposition.

Racial Poisons, Eugenics, and Sanitation

Preventive eugenics was not the whole of eugenics in Latin America. Eugenics had several manifestations, particularly in the racial-sexual sphere. But as we begin to uncover the insistent association of eugenics with sanitation, social hygiene, mental hygiene, or the hygiene of the reproductive cells, we begin also to understand some of the features that set eugenics apart in Latin countries, as well as the continued appeal of a medical-technical movement long after it

63. Eduardo Pradel Hanecuwicz, "Matrimonio y eugenesia" (Chile, 1926), Tesis Universitarias 50:42.

had been anathematized as morally and scientifically unacceptable. To many Latin American doctors, *their* eugenics stood for something different from that practiced in the United States or Germany. Various names for this eugenics suggest themselves to the historian: "preventive eugenics," "social eugenics," "eugenics and social medicine," "eugenic hygiene."[64] But whatever the name, it meant a eugenics that linked a sanitary environment to racial health. Since these sanitation dimensions of eugenics are rarely discussed in histories of eugenics, and since they challenge the typical understanding of eugenics, they deserve their own analysis.

A central factor in the Lamarckian outlook on preventive eugenics, as we have seen, was the idea of "racial poisons," a term eugenists used to refer to such things as alcohol, nicotine, morphine, venereal diseases, and other drugs and infections. These poisons were called "racial" because, though the habits and diseases were often first acquired or experienced in one individual's lifetime, they were believed to lead to permanent, hereditary degenerations that in the long run could affect entire populations or nations. The eugenists had in mind functionally produced modifications caused by, for example, "soaking the entire organism for years in the poison of syphilis," as Saleeby phrased it.[65] Avoidance of sexual "contaminations" was therefore a logical social recommendation derived from eugenic science.

Historians have tended to make little of the term or the idea of racial poisons, mainly because the mainline eugenics movements rejected such Lamarckian thinking.[66] To Latin Americans, however, control of racial poisons was a characteristic strategy that gave the movement its identity. It meant merging eugenics with preventive

64. For reasons developed in this chapter, I use the term "preventive eugenics."
65. Caleb William Saleeby, "Racial Poison," *Eugenics Review* 2 (April 1910–January 1911): 30–52.
66. Paul Weindling devotes several pages to the notion of racial poisons in the pre-eugenic era in Germany; see his *Health, Race, and German Politics between National Unification and Nazism, 1870–1945* (Cambridge: Cambridge University Press, 1989), pp. 170–88. The fate of Saleeby, the British eugenist who claimed to have coined the term in 1907 and whose ideas closely paralleled the Latin Americans', is instructive. His views were derided by Karl Pearson as completely "unscientific," and Saleeby found himself increasingly marginalized in British eugenics circles. He was eventually voted out of elective office in the council of the British Eugenics Education Society, and his offers to present papers were rebuffed. See G. R. Searle, *Eugenics and Politics in Britain, 1900–1914* (Leyden: Nordhoff International, 1976), pp. 17–19.

sanitation or expanding preventive sanitation to include the sanitation of human heredity. Of course, most of the self-styled eugenists in Latin America adopted their social policies with little regard to the niceties of genetic science. Many were clinical doctors unversed in experimental biology and concerned mainly with identifying the signs of hereditary "degeneracy" and "unfitness" in their patients, a medical exercise that deeply reflected their racial, gender, and class biases. Nevertheless, in so far as eugenics was a social movement that took its identity from science it is legitimate to ask whether and how different theories became imbued with different social values. Was a "soft" theory of inheritance correlated with "soft" policies, that is, environmental rather than biological ones? In which political circumstances? It is especially important to examine this question in relation to neo-Lamarckism, since social Lamarckism has been left out of history, and with it a systematic analysis of its associated political projects.[67]

We have seen that many eugenists of a Weismann-Mendelian persuasion interpreted genetics to mean that heredity prevailed over the environment and that only a policy devoted to breeding—to regulating the production of innate fitness—was "eugenic." This interpretation led very often to something of a disjunction between eugenics and traditional public-health or social reforms, since medical care of the sick and social welfare measures were seen as needlessly interfering with natural selection and the elimination of the unfit. Many eugenists even recommended eugenics as a kind of alternative to traditional medicine. The British scientist Karl Pearson went much further; to him, writes Kevles, "the eight-hour day, free medical advice, and reductions in infant mortality encouraged an increase in unemployables, degenerates, and physical and mental weaklings."[68] Social-medical reforms were, in the circumstances, tantamount to encouraging the formation of an increasingly "dysgenic" population, since it was also argued that the poor unfit bred faster than the middle-class fit. Pearson concluded that long-term

67. The various political projects of Darwinism have of course been much studied. For a brief discussion of social Lamarckism, see Nancy Leys Stepan, "Nature's Pruning Hook: War, Race, and Evolution, 1914–1918," in *The Political Culture of Modern Britain*, ed. J. M. W. Bean (London: Hamish Hamilton, 1987), pp. 129–45.

68. Daniel J. Kevles, *In the Name of Eugenics: Genetics and the Uses of Human Heredity* (Cambridge: Harvard University Press, 1985), pp. 34–45.

genetic improvement could therefore come about only by attention to human breeding itself. His hard-nosed attitude toward public-health reforms naturally enough irritated traditional medical-health officers, for whom environmental reforms defined their mission and their professional identity.[69]

This disjunction between public health and eugenics was often lacking in Latin America. The eugenists were uncomfortable with the distinction between eugenics and the environment, and claimed that the amelioration of the human race depended on heredity *and* environment. One of the appeals of neo-Lamarckism was precisely that a blurring of the distinction between nature and nurture kept a place for purposive social action and moral choice. Neo-Lamarckism lent itself, therefore, to a particular form of "environmental melior-ism." Although this view was by no means the only one that could be derived from Lamarckian premises, Léonard notes of French eu-genics that the doctors in France in the 1920s had many reasons for preferring to interpret neo-Lamarckism in this melioristic fashion, since it legitimated hygiene, dietetics, puericulture, and preventive medicine. The pronatalism of doctors in France supported a gener-alized concern for improving the conditions surrounding reproduc-tion, rather than for reducing the reproduction of the unfit. Uncer-tainty about the laws of heredity was a further incentive for what Léonard calls "prudent genetics."[70] The British Lamarckian and eu-genist Caleb William Saleeby, whose concept of racial poisons was in many respects the same as that of the Latin Americans, coined the term "preventive eugenics" for that portion of the social program of eugenics dealing with the eradication of racial poisons and venereal disease. Preventive eugenics was then distinguished from "positive" eugenics, which was concerned with providing incentives for the reproduction of the fit, and from "negative" eugenics, designed to

69. The legislative means by which the human race would be improved was un-clear; some kind of social incentive, such as a family allowance for the fit, was often discussed. The divergence between the traditional physicians in public health and sanitation and the eugenists, though real enough, also disguised some common-alities. Some historians suggest seeing the two groups as embracing two different forms of biological engineering, whose common goal, says Gary Wersky, was to preserve the social order (*The Visible College* [London: Allen Lane, 1978], p. 30).

70. Léonard, "Eugénisme et Darwinisme" [note 51], p. 193.

control or prevent the reproduction of the unfit.[71] It was a set of distinctions many Latin Americans liked.[72]

Extracting a sanitation-oriented, meliorist meaning from genetics in this way was essentially a political matter. Like Weismannism, neo-Lamarckism offered a number of interpretive possibilities, all of which seemed logical and/or natural conclusions of science. A positive view of the possibility of hereditary improvement through reforms of the environment in which human beings lived could be countered by the pessimistic view that the accumulated burdens of past negative environmental influences had created a thoroughly degenerate heredity that was difficult to improve rapidly. Such an interpretation could support a highly racist view of populations and drastic actions to curtail the breeding of degenerates and exclude "unfit" individuals and types from the national body. Which view prevailed was determined by an interplay of political, social, and other factors. The politics of science in specific circumstances was the critical factor.[73]

In Brazil and Argentina, the threats of radical working-class challenges to the political system—challenges that had led to strikes, protests, and severe repression on the part of the authorities in the first two decades of the century—had by the 1920s been contained; in comparison with the previous decade, the period was, relatively speaking, one of lowered conflict over the terms of the social contract. The immediate postwar years were therefore ones of some optimism concerning the possibility of social improvement and "normalization" of the nation through the reform of the medical-urban-sanitary environment. This view seemed to provide a political space for the use of medically inspired eugenic ideas that involved no radical revisioning of class relations. Later, in the more turbulent 1930s, as class conflicts intensified, more extreme and racialized eugenics emerged.

Structurally and scientifically, too, in the 1920s the neo-Lamarck-

71. See the report on the lecture by Caleb W. Saleeby, titled "Imperial Eugenics," in *Eugenics Review* 17 (April 1915–January 1916): 160.

72. Here I am drawing attention not merely to a parallel with Saleeby's terminology and ideas but to their actual adoption by some Latin Americans. See, for example, the direct reference to Saleeby's ideas in Astoquiza Sazzo, *Eugenesia* (Valparaiso: Pacífico, 1938), p. 2. Many Latin Americans tended to associate Saleeby primarily with "preventive eugenics," which was their own interest. Saleeby actually thought negative eugenics crucial.

73. On this point see Bowler, *The Eclipse of Darwinism* [note 13], p. 101.

ian outlook in eugenics was broadly congruent with the sanitation sciences, which had only recently established themselves at the center of programs of improvement. These sciences had significant ideological meanings on which eugenics could also draw and which worked to pull eugenics at first in a sanitation-oriented, reformist direction. This ideological role for sanitation derived in part from the very potency of racist and climatic explanations of degeneration in European science, explanations that haunted Latin American intellectuals. In the early part of the twentieth century, many Latin American hygienists turned to the gains made in sanitation to challenge the traditional view that race and climate in Latin America combined to produce degraded and backward nations. This challenge to conventional wisdom was especially noticeable in Brazil, where the supposed "tropicality" and "degeneracy" of the country's mixed-race population were sensitive subjects. Moreover, as medicine expanded, it included many individuals whose own racial identities were not "pure." Public hygiene was therefore viewed as a way of rescuing the country from racial and climatic "degeneracy." For instance, some hygienists denied that Brazil's tropical environment per se was hostile to the white race or caused specific diseases, as defined by the new field of tropical medicine. A Brazilian thesis of white acclimatization in the tropics emerged in the work of doctors, running counter to the common European views that for climatic reasons the white race was unable to work and thrive in extreme heat short of stringent medical and racial precautions and that the low productivity and reproductivity of the Brazilians were due to permanent features of climate and race. In his early books, *My Country, My People* and the more technical work *Hygiene*, Afrânio Peixoto, the professor of public hygiene in the Rio Medical School, criticized European medical scientists for defaming the Brazilian climate and denied the existence of tropical diseases.[74] At work within medicine was an effort to resist outside claims of inherent Brazilian degeneracy and to reclaim the country's original identity as a site of tropical salubrity.[75] Such a thesis of white acclimatization and clima-

74. Afrânio Peixoto, *Minha terra, minha gente* (São Paulo: Francisco Alves, 1916), esp. pp. 207–8, and *Hygiene* (Rio de Janeiro: Francisco Alves, 1917), pp. 68–69; see also Thomas E. Skidmore, *Black into White: Race and Nationality in Brazilian Thought* (New York: Oxford University Press, 1974).

75. On the shift in attitude toward the salubrity of the tropics in the mid–nineteenth century, see Donald Cooper, "Brazil's Long Fight against Epidemic Disease,

tic health provided the perfect scientific rationale for white immigration, something the European-oriented elites actively desired in the hope of "whitening" Brazil's population.[76]

Given this racialized context, we can understand the enthusiasm of many Latin American physicians for the new bacteriological and microbiological sciences when they were introduced at the end of the nineteenth century and the start of the twentieth. These sciences were seen to offer practical solutions to epidemic disease as well as rebuttals to the thesis of the inevitability of Latin American degeneration and racial ill health.[77] Rebuilding the cities, moving the middle classes to healthy districts, setting up new public-health and bacteriological laboratories, "sanitizing" the poor by compulsory vaccination and other public-health measures—all were part of the repertoire of sanitation policies that had been adopted in many Latin American countries by the time eugenics made its appearance. Admittedly many of these measures were ineffectual, even misplaced and misguided, driven as much by the desire to seal off and "fumigate" centers of supposed social and medical contamination as by genuine humanitarian impulses; but one result of the emphasis on sanitation was the merging of eugenics in social hygiene, or the eugenization of public health.

In fact, many hygienists initially interpreted the new eugenics as simply a new branch of traditional public hygiene. Hence, for instance, the insistence by Olegario de Mouro, vice-president of the São Paulo Eugenics Society, that "to sanitize *is* to eugenize" ("sanear é eugenizar"). He maintained that sanitation was the same thing that some people called "eugenics," adding that for public understanding, it was better to call it santitation, though the word "eugenics" was better "scientifically." He himself equated them as follows: "Saneamento-eugenia é ordem e progresso" ("Sanitation-eugenics is order and progress").[78] This broad congruence between eugenics and sanitation was reflected in many other Latin American movements

1847–1901," *Bulletin of the New York Acadamy of Medicine* 51 (1975): 672–96, where he shows how yellow fever and cholera epidemics of the mid–nineteenth century helped crystallize the image of Brazil as essentially unhealthy.

76. "Whitening" via European immigration was a process sought by the elite in many other Latin American countries in the nineteenth and twentieth centuries. This point is discussed further in Chapter 5.

77. Nancy Stepan, *Beginnings of Brazilian Science: Oswaldo Cruz, Medical Research and Policy, 1890–1930* (New York: Science History Publications, 1976), p. 58.

78. Olegario de Moura, "Saneamento-eugenía-civilização," *Annães de Eugenía* (São Paulo: Sociedade Eugénica de São Paulo, Revista do Brasil, 1919), p. 83.

as well. In Argentina, in a much-cited work, Jorge A. Frías referred to "the methods of positive eugenics for improving the state of public health, combating all sorts of epidemics and endemics—the battle against malaria, tuberculosis, cancer, plagues, venereal infections, alcoholism." At times the public-health branch of eugenics was referred to as "indirect eugenic methods."[79]

Although the causes embraced by the Mendelians and the neo-Lamarckian eugenists were sometimes similar, the style of their eugenics was somewhat different and at times led the eugenists to distinctive or contrary conclusions. The Mendelians often argued, as we have seen, that medical care and welfare provisions caused natural selection to lose much of its force, as the unfit were increasingly being allowed to survive and pass on their poor qualities to future generations. A deliberate "eugenic" social selection of the fit then became the modern answer, as it were, to the decline of natural selection.

But, as the British K. E. Trounson had said, Brazilian eugenists tended to neglect both natural and social selection. Instead, Latin Americans generally emphasized, as Saleeby did, the extended scope of action of racial poisons in the modern world and the need to carry out a concerted attack on them. The attitudes toward social reform were therefore often subtly different in the two kinds of eugenics movements. Leonard Darwin, president of the Eugenics Education Society in England, did not deny the value of sanitation, but he made it clear that the specific terrain of eugenics, in terms of its scientific rationale and its practical policies, was indeed distinct from that of traditional public health.[80] Any merger of the two was wrong scientifically and practically, because it would diminish the force of the new eugenic idea. To the Latin Americans, the opposite was true: the elimination of racial poisons helped define the movement. To a neo-Lamarckian, alcoholism, poor living conditions, and work fatigue were eugenic issues precisely because they were both causes and symptoms of hereditary ills and because the cycle of causes could be interrupted by social, moral, and medical action. Since the neo-Lamarckian style of eugenics kept open the possibility of "regeneration" as the answer to the fear of racial "degeneration," its approach allowed a fusion of moral and scientific language. Poverty,

79. Frías, El matrimonio [note 4], pp. 149–50.
80. Leonard Darwin, The Need for Eugenic Reform (New York: Appleton, 1926), pp. 83–93.

venereal diseases, and alcoholism could then be interpreted as products of both social conditions and immoral behavior.

As in France, the neo-Lamarckian outlook of the eugenists allowed alliances to be forged between the eugenists and the more broadly defined sanitation and public-hygiene organizations. In Brazil, for instance, Lamarckian eugenics brought in such allies from the rural-sanitation movement as Belisário Penna, whose long journey by horseback in 1913 among the diseased populations of the northeastern states of Brazil had made him a crusader for rural health. As Kehl's eventual father-in-law, Penna was a most useful and strategic addition to eugenics, capable of winning support from like-minded hygienists. Other allies were recruited from the pro-sanitation and nationalistic leagues that had sprouted in Brazil before and after World War I. There was considerable overlap in membership and style of discourse between the Nationalist League of São Paulo and the São Paulo Eugenics Society; indeed, the president of the second, Arnaldo Vieira de Carvalho, was the vice president of the first. To the intelligentsia, already predisposed to promote sanitation as a cure-all for Latin America's woes, eugenics appealed as a kind of scientific extension and modernization of the work of such heroic figures as Oswaldo Cruz and Carlos Chagas, and as a way of reducing the extraordinarily high infant-mortality rates and the sickly condition of the masses. Even the promotion of sports and physical fitness could be claimed to be eugenic because they "improved the race." Eugenics had become a metaphor for health itself.

The neo-Lamarckian style of Latin eugenics was represented in its purest form, perhaps, in the eugenic antialcohol campaigns of the 1920s. Alcoholism was connected to puericulture and eugenics because it was believed, as we have seen, that the consumption of alcohol over long periods of time resulted in hereditary defects in offspring. Most physicians, of course, reasoned backward—from the supposed evidences of idiocy, epilepsy, mental illness, juvenile delinquency, and other pathologies to the existence of a family history of alcoholism. Sorting out what was a biological form of inheritance from what was a social inheritance, or what was genetic inheritance from what was "congenital" (i.e., a defect arising in the process of birth itself, perhaps via toxins in the mother's bloodstream, but not affecting the genetic makeup) was of course virtually impossible given the hereditary outlook of the doctors. From a practical point of view, attacking the consumption of alcohol and moralizing about social habits became a logical step in eugenics. It also allowed the eugenists to draw boundaries between acceptable and unacceptable social behaviors. Since these boundaries also separated the poor from the middle class, the manual workers from the elite, and the white segments of the population from the dark, the eugenists' attack on racial poisons also reelaborated notions of race and set new terms by which the internal boundaries between peoples were to be understood.[81] While the puericulture-eugenists conceptualized women as primarily reproductive beings for whom "protection" and scientific obstetrics were the appropriate medical responses, they conceptualized men as above all sexual beings whose sexuality itself could cause degeneration. Eugenists singled out poor, urban, working-class males as especially prone to undisciplined sexuality and drunkenness; for this reason, much of the antialcohol rhetoric associated with the eugenics-puericulture movement was directed most specifically against them.

Experimental evidence was often cited to prove the effects of racial poisons. Whereas in England Pearson and other strict eugenists insisted that alcoholism had nothing to do with heredity, the Latin Americans were wont to quote whatever scientific facts they could find to support the view that racial poisons did indeed cause deterioration over several generations.[82] They cited, for instance, Valentin Magnan's laboratory studies on the deleterious effects of intoxicants, which had resulted in the prohibition of absinthe in most European countries by 1918.[83] It is not surprising, given the context, that the first scientific task Enrique Beltrán approached as a fledgling biologist in Mexico in the 1920s was to test the possible effects of pulque, the intoxicating drink favored by the Mexican poor, on

81. For the notion of internal boundaries, see Ann Laura Stoler, "Making the Empire Respectable: Race and Sexual Morality in Twentieth-Century Colonial Cultures," *American Ethnologist* 16 (1989): 634–60.

82. See Kevles, *In the Name of Eugenics* [note 68], p. 105.

83. See Robert A. Nye, *Crime, Madness, and Politics in Modern France: The Medical Concept of National Decline* (Princeton, N.J.: Princeton University Press, 1984), p. 123. The damaging effects of alcohol on heredity was not only a French and Latin American concern; Nazi doctors studied the effects of alcohol on the germ plasm, and in 1937 the sale of alcohol to minors was restricted in Germany. In the United States, too, the control of alcohol was at times part of eugenics. On Germany, see Robert N. Proctor, *Racial Hygiene: Medicine under the Nazis* (Cambridge: Harvard University Press, 1988), pp. 238–41; on the United States, see the occasional references to alcoholism in Kevles, *In the Name of Eugenics* [note 68], e.g., p. 64.

laboratory animals.[84] A few years later, the first action taken by the Technical Consultative Committee of the Mexican Eugenics Society was to investigate whether intoxicants were causes of "racial decay."[85]

Long viewed as a social and moral evil in itself, especially of the poor (and, in much of Latin America, racially mixed) population, alcoholism was now reformulated as an "enemy of the race" because the vice supposedly caused hereditary conditions linked to crime, juvenile delinquency, prostitution, and mental illness and because its effects were felt for generations afterward.[86] The Brazilian hygienist and eugenist Afrânio Peixoto, for example, campaigned against alcohol because he said it caused the children to be defective, predisposed from infancy to meningitis, convulsions, mental deficiency, madness, and crime.[87] The League of Mental Hygiene took the hereditary effects of alcohol as its special concern, lecturing the public about the evils of intoxicants, which were presented as having a "sterilizing" influence on the masses by causing low reproductive rates, high mortality, and hereditary taint. In an article in *Brasil-Médico* in 1929, Francisco Prisco commented on the reduction in the working population caused by alcohol, and on its consequences for the children who were born.[88] The League promoted "antialcohol" weeks in 1927, 1928, 1929, and 1931, featuring public addresses and radio talks by such well-known figures as Juliano Moreira, considered to be the father of psychiatry in Brazil. In October 1929 the league created a new section devoted specifically to agitating against alcoholism and to stimulating public interest and financial support for their work. American-style prohibition, taxes on imported and nationally produced alcohol, special reformatories for the "inveterate drunkard," all were discussed and promoted by the league as eugenic measures. In Mexico, the state of Veracruz went further and

84. Beltrán, "Cándido Bolívar Pieltain" [note 21], p. 9.
85. *Boletín de la Sociedad Eugénica Mexicana* 3 (September 1, 1932): 2.
86. For a typical statement, see the eugenics pamphlet by Juan Astorquiza Sazzo, Jr., *Eugenesia* (Valparaiso: Droguería del Pacífico, 1938), in which the author cited numerous, mainly French sources on the effect of alcohol on the "germinative protoplasm of procreation" and therefore descendants.
87. Afrânio Peixoto, *Criminología* (São Paulo: Editora Nacional, 1936), pp. 209–11.
88. Francisco Prisco, "Alcoolismo," *Brasil-Médico* 43 (1929): 801–5.

experimented with prohibition for many of the same hygienic and eugenic reasons.[89]

A Contestation over Meaning: The Attack on Neo-Lamarckism

To a large extent the Latin American eugenists' assumptions were unconsciously rather than consciously neo-Lamarckian. For this reason disputes arose only rarely about the scientific bases of eugenics. But when they did, they were very revealing about the scientific-social constructions many physicians had put upon eugenics.

One place where such a dispute surfaced was Brazil. By the second half of the 1920s, a new generation of biological scientists had begun to emerge, most of them employed in agricultural rather than medical institutions and many of them beginning to become knowledgeable about the scientific differences between Anglo-Saxon Mendelism and Latin neo-Lamarckism. Mendelism had been consolidated in the United States, which was fast emerging as a leader in science and as a new pole of attraction for Latin American students seeking training abroad. Moreover, progressive circles, such as those surrounding the anthropologist Franz Boas, were championing antiracist positions, which also affected some members of the new generation of social and biological scientists in Brazil. Some of these new Mendelians turned their critical eye on the neo-Lamarckian eugenics movement, which they believed was out of step with modern views.

Of the Mendelian critics, the anthropologist Edgar Roquette-Pinto, director of the National Museum of Anthropology in Rio de Janeiro between 1916 and 1936, was perhaps the most important because of his role as president of the First Brazilian Eugenics Congress, held in 1929. In a book of essays published two years before the congress, Roquette-Pinto had defined eugenics as a method of artifical selection of human heredity based on three components of modern genetics—cytology, biometry, and experimental biology.[90]

89. This ban was part of the eugenics law passed by the state of Veracruz in 1932; since the law also introduced extreme reproductive measures, I analyze it in Chapter 4, on eugenics and reproduction.

90. Edgar Roquette-Pinto, *Seixos rolados (Estudos brasileiros)* (Rio de Janeiro: n.p., 1927).

By 1928 he was citing Mendelian geneticists (such as the extremist Charles Davenport) in support of the position that "every educated person knows that, actually, the celebrated 'influence of the environment' has been reduced to very restricted limits." "The majority of biologists," he commented, "do not believe that the environment is capable of influencing hereditary characters, all of which are dependent on the germ plasm. The environment, it is currently believed, modifies only the somatoplasm, the part of living things that does not become part of inheritance."[91] Roquette-Pinto later expressed the hope that the confusion between eugenics and sanitation, much in evidence at the eugenics congress in 1929, would in the future be cleared up.

A second locus of Mendelian genetics was the Agricultural School at Piracicaba, where Carlos Teixeira Mendes was a professor; his interest in plant breeding may have explained his early adoption of Mendelism and the new science of hybridization. In a period when institutions in Brazil with a practical bent were rapidly developing, and in a state (São Paulo) where the need to expand agricultural production was felt most strongly, a Mendelian science of hybridization provided techniques for the improvement of export crops. In 1918 Teixeira Mendes gave the first lectures in Brazil on Mendelian genetics, in his own department and in the department of "zootechnics" headed by Dr. Octavio Domingues.[92] Domingues also became an important disseminator of Mendelian genetics in Brazil, and, if not an original experimentalist, he was an interesting figure in the Brazilian eugenics movement.

As a member of the American Genetics Association and the Eugenics Education Society of Great Britain, Domingues held to a strictly Mendelian outlook. His eugenic texts, such as *Heredity in the Face of Education*, published in 1929, were among the first books in Brazil to review systematically and in an up-to-date fashion North American, British, and European genetics for scientists and the general reading public (necessarily small in Brazil). Domingues cited, among others, Francis Galton, Karl Pearson, R. C. Punnett, Thomas Hunt Morgan, Charles Davenport, W. E. Castle, Edwin

91. Edgar Roquette-Pinto, *Ensaios de antropología brasileiro* (1933; Rio de Janeiro: Editora Nacional, 1978), p. 35.
92. Only many years later was Mendelian genetics used systematically for improving coffee, corn, tobacco, and similar crops in the state.

G. Conklin, and H. S. Jennings, as well as the French biologists Lucien Cuénot and Emile Guyenot.[93]

In his analyses of contemporary genetic theory, Domingues criticized the neo-Lamarckism of his fellow eugenists, calling it a deformation of science caused by too great a dependency on French biology, though he noted that even among French scientists one could find critics of Lamarck, citing Cuénot as an example. In 1930 he complained in the Brazilian journal *Bulletin of Eugenics* that, with few exceptions, Brazilians were ignorant of (Mendelian) genetics, and as late as 1936 he claimed that few Brazilians had ever heard of the founder of modern chromosome theory, Thomas Hunt Morgan.[94] Domingues lamented that his fellow eugenists were "following an erroneous path, confusing eugenics with individual and social hygiene, with gymnastics, individual physical development, with sports—subjects that ally them with the science of Galton, but that are not really eugenics."[95] He reiterated his warning seven years later, implying that the eugenists had not learned their lesson: "Among us, when our hygienists pride themselves on recommending cleanliness, good hygienic habits, abstinence from alcohol, smoking, or other stupefactants, or when they [promote] national gymnastics, they make these recommendations thinking that what a person acquires in a lifetime is transmitted to offspring. Therefore, one way to improve the race genetically is to adopt these measures, so that in a few generations our people will be transformed into pure Greeks—with beautiful bodies and physiognomies."[96] Domingues countered this notion of inheritance with a strictly Mendelian one, distinguishing biological inheritance from social inheritance and calling for a program of "true" eugenics and eutechnics (or general sanitation properly understood) to create a healthy social environment in which the genetically fit could thrive.

On these points Domingues was supported by the young André Dreyfus, later one of the pioneers of Mendelian genetics in Brazil at

93. Octavio Domingues, *Hereditariedade e eugenía: Suas bases, suas teorias, suas applicações práticas* (Rio de Janeiro: Civilização Brasileira, 1936), and *Eugenía: Seus propósitos, suas bases, seus meios* (São Paulo: Editora Nacional, 1942).

94. Octavio Domingues, "Os programmas de ensino e a genética," *Boletim de Eugenía* 9(92) (1930): 50–51, and *Hereditariedade e eugenía* [note 93], pp. 145–50.

95. Octavio Domingues, *A hereditariedade em face de educação* (São Paulo: Melhoramentos, 1929), p. 139.

96. Domingues, *Hereditariedade e eugenía* [note 93], p. 147.

the University of São Paulo. In the 1920s he too tried to put right what he saw as errors in the ideas of his fellow biologists and physicians. At the First Brazilian Eugenics Congress in 1929 in Rio, Dreyfus pointed out that Mendelian laws and their experimental confirmation had given genetics an entirely new orientation. He noted that alternatives such as Galton's law of ancestral inheritance, which eugenists repeatedly cited, were now taken seriously only by researchers "distant from the positive results of genetics." All efforts to confirm Lamarckian notions experimentally had failed, he said, and as a result, the belief of "various eugenists that a favorable environment, good food, and instruction will be able to influence the hereditary patrimony" had "sadly to be abandoned."[97] In 1943 Dreyfus invited the Russian-born geneticist Theodosius Dobzhansky to Brazil to train what became the first group of researchers to experiment on Drosophila fruit flies. The fact that two years later Dreyfus felt it necessary to repeat his censure of neo-Lamarckian inheritance suggests the extraordinary persistence of the belief in the transmission of acquired characters.[98]

Few of these scientific critics wanted to give up eugenics entirely, but they wanted to provide it with a more solid foundation. Their scientific critique of neo-Lamarckian genetics became a matter of public notice at the First Brazilian Eugenics Congress of 1929, where it took many of the eugenists by surprise. The physician Levi Carneiro, presiding over the section on education and legislation, spoke directly to the issue of the scientific bases of eugenics; in his view, the denial of neo-Lamarckian heredity negated the importance of alcohol and venereal diseases for racial (i.e., hereditary) improvement. Carneiro spoke for many of his fellow eugenists when he defended neo-Lamarckian inheritance (citing Charles Richet and Frédéric Houssay), but he was uncertain enough of his grounds to admit that the influence of the milieu on the germ plasm was not entirely established. But Carneiro clearly understood the critics to mean that the denial of the transmission of acquired characters called into question the scientific rationale of such things as the antialcohol

97. André Dreyfus, "O estado actual do problema de hereditariedade," in Primeiro Congresso Brasileiro de Eugenia, Actos e Trabalhos (Rio de Janeiro, 1929), pp. 87–97.

98. André Dreyfus, "Curso de genética, com aplicação a orquidología," Boletim do Círculo Paulista de Orquidófilos 2 (1945): 51–58, 69–78, 89–102, 109–17, 125–32, 141–46, 157–64.

campaigns with which the League of Mental Hygiene was so closely identified. Understandably, the founder of the league, Gustavo Reidel, continued to reserve his opinion on the applicability of Mendelian laws to the human species, maintaining that as far as he was concerned, mental discord and mental illness had direct hereditary effects on offspring, so that the eugenic program of mental hygiene was fully justified.[99]

The effect of the Mendelian critique on neo-Lamarckian eugenics can perhaps be seen most strikingly in the writings of the tireless promotor of Brazilian eugenics, Renato Kehl. By the late 1920s Kehl had begun to turn in a more racist and conservative direction. He now found irritating what had once been an advantage; namely, the confusion in the public mind between eugenics and sanitation. As he later explained, allies from the sanitation movements had been useful at the beginning of the eugenics campaign, when public understanding of eugenics was slight and when he himself, as he admitted, was not entirely clear about the distinction between sanitation and eugenics.[100] But when the elite embraced personal hygiene, physical excercise, and organized sport as "eugenic," Kehl began to protest that ordinary hygiene could not improve the hereditary stock of Brazil; it certainly did not, in his view, begin to address the real racial-eugenic problems of the nation. Yet even Kehl found it hard to abandon the Lamarckian, preventive notion of eugenics that had defined the movement in Brazil for so long. By 1929 he was ready to concede that syphilis and tuberculosis did not cause hereditary conditions, as he had previously believed, but caused only congenital damage limited to a single generation. He agreed, that is, that in these cases the "racial" poison did not permanently modify the reproductive material. But in the *Lessons in Eugenics* Kehl's review of theories of heredity continued to be eclectic, evidence of the state of flux in hereditary theory in Latin American circles. The neo-Lamarckism of Edward Drinker Cope, the neo-Darwinism of Weismann, the preadaptationism of Cuénot, the mutationism of De Vries, and the chromosome theory of Morgan—all were presented to the Brazilian reader, with no discrimination

99. Levi Carneiro, "Educação e eugenía," in Primeiro Congresso Brasileiro de Eugeniá, *Actos e Trabalhos* (Rio de Janeiro, 1929), p. 112.

100. Kehl, *Lições de eugenía* [note 59], p. 22, and *Porque sou eugenista* (Rio de Janeiro: Francisco Alves, 1937), p. 147.

among them. Moreover, Kehl's use of the term "eugenismo" (euge-nism) to describe *all* the activities that aided eugenics, including edu-cation, sanitation, sports, legislation, and hygiene, blurred the very distinction he said he now sought to draw *between* eugenics and sani-tation, or "eutechnics."[101] The Mendelian attack on Lamarckism *and* eugenics had, for the moment, failed to dislodge the neo-Lamarck-ian outlook of most of the eugenists.

Racial Poisons and Social Meanings

In the 1930s, many of the countries of Latin America began to experience the effects of the depression and entered a period of con-siderable political turmoil, with a resultant turn to right-wing and conservative politics. Yet the preventive eugenics of the 1920s also remained a lasting feature of the Latin style of eugenics. In Brazil, for example, when new social security measures—unemployment benefits, pensions, protective labor legislation—were introduced by the new Ministry of Labor in the 1930s, the eugenists greeted them as significant contributions to "racial improvement." Kehl's notion of "eugenismo," directed toward making the environment "fit for reproduction," had its counterparts in the ideologically different countries of Mexico and Argentina. In 1932 the Mexican eugenist Saavedra called for general hygiene, antialcohol campaigns, a battle against toximanias, sports education, the regulation of work, the prohibition of women's work in certain industries or at certain "dangerous" times (e.g., at night), a minimum-wage law, and a re-duction in the cost of living.

At times the admiration expressed by self-styled eugenists for so-cial and worker legislation was a matter of *faute de mieux*—a reflec-tion of the lack of anything more obviously specifically eugenic to praise in national legislation. Moreover, since much of the welfare legislation was more often than not completely ineffective, because it was never actually implemented, the eugenists' preventive eu-genics was more rhetorical than real. Preventive eugenics generated a set of cultural prescriptions that operated as conscious and uncon-

101. Kehl, *Porque sou eugenista* [note 100], pp. 46–47; in 1937 Kehl also still made use of the concept of blastophthoric disorders, especially with reference to the dam-age caused by alcohol in reproduction.

scious sanctions concerning behavior. It put forward an extremely reductive and inadequate framework for interpreting the medical and social problems of what were in most cases very poor populations—inadequate because in Latin America, where child labor was commonplace, infant and maternal mortality and morbidity from preventable endemic illnesses were extremely high, and the conditions of labor were extraordinarily bad, the hereditary aspects of poverty and disease were minor in comparison with the economic and political ones. Preventive eugenics treated the highly complex social results of misery and poverty with biological metaphors of heredity and race improvement. The focus on the supposedly permanent degenerations caused in human populations by racial poisons led to an emphasis on the need for state programs of sanitary registration and control of the sickly, undernourished, and badly housed poor; to the use of the techniques of "mental hygiene" for the eugenization of "undisciplined" workers as a way to achieve their "purification"; to an exhortation to moral virtue as the centerpiece of sanitary education.

By structuring the perceptions of ill health in terms of hereditary and racial "degeneration," the eugenists moved their considerations from the political and economic spheres to the hereditary. In this respect, the preventive eugenics described in this chapter, though distinctive in comparative terms, had strategically much in common with eugenics movements in other parts of the world.

4

"Matrimonial Eugenics": Gender and the Construction of Negative Eugenics

The most notorious techniques introduced by eugenists to "improve the race" involved the direct prevention of human reproduction. When we think of eugenics, we think of compulsory human sterilization, compulsory sexual segregation, and even euthanasia. Measures such as these were justified by eugenists in various parts of the world as effective measures to eradicate bad heredity in human populations and thereby to ensure the continued progress of human society. A negative eugenics was thus defined. Eugenists thought of human reproduction not as an individual activity and as an outcome of human sexuality but as a collective responsibility and a producer of good or bad heredity. Eugenists therefore were engaged in a radical revision of the meaning of sexual reproduction to society, and of the individual right to that reproduction.

Nearly all histories of eugenics take negative reproductive eugenics as central to the movement. But by these criteria, Latin Americans were outside eugenics; with rare (but telling) exceptions, sterilization, abortion, and birth control were not legalized as eugenic measures, and therefore they did not define the field. Nevertheless, particularly in the 1930s, the Latin American eugenists proposed their own form of negative reproductive eugenics, a form that once again tends to be overlooked in histories of eugenics. As an Argentinian doctor put it, society had to be concerned not just with "impeding the acquisition of degenerate characters that were transmissible by heredity," in the preventive fashion described in the last chapter, but with actually "controlling the marriages between the defective and degenerate".[1] The Latin Americans asked themselves whether a negative eugenics of reproduction and marriage could be constructed which was nonetheless compatible with the very real political and other constraints that Latin American society placed on a radical refiguration of sexuality and reproduction. They answered that it could—that there could be a "Christian" view of eugenics.[2] The result was a special form of negative or "matrimonial eugenics," setting new scientific-hereditary norms and controls over reproduction, without encompassing radical surgical methods.

Elements of this matrimonial eugenics formed part of eugenics in other parts of the world.[3] For example, the prenuptial medical tests and certificates that were important components of matrimonial eugenics in Latin America were also made compulsory by several legislatures in the United States. But whereas in the United States these tests were viewed as, strictly speaking, only supplements to other eugenic policies, and not always effective ones at that, in Latin America they were central aspects of a wider discourse about gender, race, and the biological identity of the nation.[4]

The Discourse of Gender, Race, and Nation

Central to this discourse was gender. Gender was important to eugenics because it was through sexual reproduction that the modification and transmission of the hereditary makeup of future generations occurred. Control of that reproduction, by direct or indirect means, therefore became an important aspect of all eugenics movements. As the social role of women was viewed as primarily repro-

1. César Escudero, "Conceptos e ideales eugénicos," *Anales de Biotipología, Eugenesia y Medicina Social* 1 (August 1, 1933): 10. Hereafter *ABEMS*.
2. Octavio V. López, "Cristianismo y eugenesia," *ABEMS* 1 (August 1, 1933): 6–7.
3. Another word used was "constructive eugenics"; see Jorge A. Frías, *El matrimonio, sus impedimentos y nulidades* (Córdoba, Argentina: El Ateneo, 1941), p. 212.
4. For a Latin American view of how to classify the various branches of eugenics, see Amanda Grossi Aninat, *Eugenesia y su legislación* (Santiago: Nacimiento, 1941), p. 56.

ductive, many eugenic policies centered on them. What this attention to women signified, politically and practically, is a matter of debate. To some historians, eugenics was by definition an antifeminist, conservative movement, because it aimed to control sexuality and confine women to a reproductive-maternal role. Others, looking at the eugenists' promotion of maternal and infant health care, sexual hygiene, and sexual education, emphasize the appeal of eugenics to reformists and the left; they suggest that in its day eugenics was a progressive force, even at times protofeminist. The involvement of women themselves in eugenics causes further interpretive confusions; one study calls eugenics "one of the least sexist fields of the day in a number of countries."[5] Clearly the gender meanings of eugenics depend on where one looks. Women did not form a unitary category, any more than did men, and eugenic policies in reproduction reflected the divisions and contradictions within gender and within social life.

Equally important to negative reproductive eugenics was race and racism, since it was through sexual unions that boundaries between races were believed to be either maintained or transgressed.[6] The word "race" was a salient part of the vocabulary of eugenics in the Latin American cases, and all the eugenics movements were preoccupied with racial questions, especially as they related to sex and reproduction. As I said earlier, the particular races that concerned the eugenists (the Latins, mulattos, mestizos, Jews, Russians, Anglo-Saxons) were not preexisting, discrete, biological entities but social-political categories or perceptions created through scientific work and the social relations of power. Any history of eugenics needs to give some account of how eugenists defined the racial ele-

5. Remark by Mark B. Adams in *The Wellborn Science: Eugenics in Germany, France, Brazil, and Russia,* ed. Mark B. Adams (New York: Oxford University Press, 1990), p. 220.

6. By far the most important demonstration of this linkage is by Gisela Bock, whose studies of Nazi eugenics show that eugenics did not mean the same thing for men as for women, or for women of different races. Female "Aryans" were defined by the eugenists as reproductive beings, and laws excluded them from certain kinds of work; women of so-called undesirable races were forcibly sterilized. Thus gender was linked to race and vice versa. See Bock, "Racism and Sexism in Nazi Germany: Motherhood, Compulsory Sterilization, and the State," *Signs* 8 (1983): 400–421. Robert N. Proctor also devotes a chapter to the special policies developed for women under National Socialism; see his *Racial Hygiene: Medicine under the Nazis* (Cambridge: Cambridge University Press, 1988), chap. 4.

ments in their country and what meaning they gave to "racial purification."

Furthermore, in the 1920s and 1930s the discourse on gender and race became increasingly linked to the discourse on the nation. Eugenics has, of course, often been linked to nationalism, which, as E. J. Hobsbawm has remarked, reached its apogee between the two world wars; but the racial and gender dimensions of this link need to be emphasized.[7] The desire to "imagine" the nation in biological terms, to "purify" the reproduction of populations to fit hereditary norms, to regulate the flow of peoples across national boundaries, to define in novel terms who could belong to the nation and who could not—all these aspects of eugenics turned on issues of gender and race, and produced intrusive proposals or prescriptions for new state policies toward individuals. Through eugenics, in short, gender and race were tied to the politics of national identity.

In Latin America the development of eugenics coincided with a post–World War I reassessment of the region's potential role in the world economy and a search for national identities that would be based on the realities of the region. Eugenics also developed at a time when the United States was becoming increasingly involved in the region and when its own identity and politics depended heavily on race and immigration. In these circumstances, many Latin American intellectuals looked inward to ask whether they too had a "race spirit" that defined them and gave them a sense of national identity comparable to that of European nations.

When they did examine themselves in this way, only too often they concluded that their countries were wanting in a true "nationhood" on which to erect a proper nationalism. To the eugenists, a true nation had a common purpose, a shared language and culture, and a homogeneous population. By these criteria, many of the elite were inclined to think that Latin American countries were not yet proper nations. They especially lacked biological coherence. Because of centuries of racial mixture and immigration—from Africa, Europe, and Asia—their peoples still formed, they believed, only "raceless masses"—radical and terrifying heterogeneities instead of biological unities. Even at their best, they were, said the Argentinian

7. E. J. Hobsbawm, *Nations and Nationalism: Programme, Myth, Reality* (Cambridge: Cambridge University Press, 1990), chap. 5.

Carlos Octavio Bunge, "mestizo-ized, indian-ized, and mulatto-ized Europeans."[8]

These were, of course, the well-known national and racial stereotypes from abroad. What the Latin Americans added to the debate about the nation was the new hereditary science. The question they asked themselves was how eugenics could play a part in creating a "true" nationality out of the peoples that made up its populations. What were the critical racial elements in their countries, and how could they be purified, unified, and homogenized? This concern for nation, identity, and homogeneity gave unity to eugenics movements that on details of political inflections, racial politics, and gender took different and even opposite positions. Thus the Mexicans praised racial hybridization as itself a form of eugenization that would help consolidate the nation around the mestizo; the Argentinians condemned racial and cultural intermixture as threats to the unity of an Argentine nationality. In both cases, the eugenists aimed to use hereditary science to produce a biologically consolidated nation.

In his influential study of nationalism, Benedict Anderson suggests we think of nations as cultural artifacts. A nation is, in his view, more than a geography, territory, government, or people; it is what Anderson calls an "imagined community." As such, a nation creates bonds of identity and belonging. As an imagined community, different individuals, ethnic groups, and races can be invited into the nation, through procedures of intermarriage, for example, or excluded from it by policies of immigration restriction and discriminatory practices. Other historical studies have also pointed to the imaginative cultural processes involved in the creation of the "nation," from the reconstruction of mythological pasts to the production of new rites and rituals around which the notion of nationality can form and be defined.[9]

Science is rarely examined as part of the project of nationalism, yet it has been a powerful discourse regulating meaning. It is the imagined community of the eugenists that interests me here—the

8. Quoted in Charles Hale, "Political and Social Ideas in Latin America, 1870–1930," in *The Cambridge History of Latin America*, ed. Leslie Bethell (Cambridge: Cambridge University Press, 1986), 4:367–441, quote on p. 400.

9. Benedict Anderson, *Imagined Communities: Reflections on the Origin and Spread of Nationalism* (London: Verso, 1986); E. J. Hobsbawm and Terence Ranger, eds., *The Invention of Tradition* (Cambridge: Cambridge University Press, 1983).

politics of its elaboration, the languages and terms used to describe it, the place of racism and sexism in the nationalist projects, and the visions of homogeneity and exclusion which a negative eugenics was designed to articulate.

The Science and Politics of Negative Reproductive Eugenics

In the delineation of the negative eugenics developed in Latin America, three factors were especially salient: the status and role of women in society, the politics of science, and the power of religion.

In Europe, eugenics coincided with a number of factors that made the reconstitution of gender crucial to it. One factor was the rise of feminism and the challenge it represented to traditional views on women's place and women's rights. Another was the increasing involvement of women in the paid work force and the ensuing changes in fertility and natality. Abortion remained illegal in almost all Western countries in the period of eugenics, but the state's ban was resisted by women determined (or forced by economic and/or psychological necessity) to control their own reproductive lives. In France, for example, the number of illegal abortions was estimated in 1937 at between 300,000 and 500,000 a year; many people believed abortions were more numerous than births.[10] Abortion and questions about fertility were linked in turn to debates about population size in relation to national strength.

Worry about changes in fertility rates, health in reproduction, and infant mortality led many women to become active in reform movements for sexual hygiene. In Germany in the 1920s, for instance, there was a sizable sex reform movement (it had an estimated membership of 150,000) that put forward a varied agenda of often conflicting goals. Mainly associated with the socialist and communist left, sex reformers demanded legalization of abortion, access to contraception, and even sterilization, all in the name of greater sexual

10. D. V. Glass, *Population: Policies and Movements in Europe* (Oxford: Clarendon Press, 1940), p. 218. The story of abortion in Europe—its legal proscription, the periods of intensification of prosecution of people involved in abortion, the concealed role of doctors and abortionists, the disguise of abortion under the rubric of necessary medical procedures, the personal costs of continued resort to clandestine abortion—is a large topic that very much needs exploring.

freedom and the modernization and medicalization of human repro-duction.[11] In the circumstances, eugenics—a secular, scientific pro-gram that dealt specifically with hereditary health in reproduction—became incorporated into the sex reform movement. Women them-selves often played prominent roles in advocating the legalization of birth control and the compulsory registration and treatment of vene-real disease. Very often, too, they accepted unthinkingly the more reprehensible racial and class biases of eugenics, thereby reflecting their own privileged status as members of the middle class. Some women found in eugenics societies a new space for social action. Even in the most medically oriented eugenics organizations, where a medical degree was a requirement for membership, women began to find opportunities for careers.[12]

This conjuncture of factors, which gave opportunities to women as subjects and authors of sexual politics within the sphere of eu-genics, was, if not entirely absent in Latin America, differently con-figured. In all three of the countries studied in this book, organized women's movements had emerged by the early twentieth century. As they expanded in the 1920s they forged links with other women's organizations in Europe and pushed to change the legal restrictions on women's rights. Yet their efforts met with great re-sistance, and the movements remained isolated, even in revolution-ary Mexico.[13] The majority of ordinary men and women saw femi-nist ideas as strange and alien interpretations of women's natural roles and needs. Mexican feminists found themselves locked in con-

11. On the German sex-hygiene movement, see Atina Grossmann, *Reforming Sex: The German Movement for Birth Control and Abortion, 1920–1950* (New York: Oxford University Press, 1995).

12. Rosaleen Love, "Alice in Eugenics-Land: Feminism and Eugenics in the Sci-entific Careers of Alice Lee and Ethel Elderton," *Annals of Science* 36 (1979): 145–58. Kevles points out in his study of Anglo-American eugenics that half of the members of the Eugenics Education Society and about a quarter of its officers were women. In the United States women were also well represented in local eugenics groups; see Daniel Kevles, *In the Name of Eugenics: Genetics and the Uses of Heredity* (New York: Knopf, 1985), p. 64. It is a mistake, then, to posit women as only "victims" of eugenics; the relation between women, gender ideology, and eugenics is more com-plex than this.

13. See June E. Hahner, *Emancipating the Female Sex: The Struggle for Women's Rights in Brazil, 1850–1940* (Durham, N.C.: Duke University Press, 1990); Marifran Carlson, *¡Feminismo!: The Women's Movement in Argentina from Its Beginnings to Eva Perón* (Chicago: Academy Chicago Publishers, 1988); and Anna Macias, *Against All Odds: The Feminist Movement in Mexico to 1940* (Westport, Conn.: Greenwood Press, 1982).

tinuous battles with the authorities and with one another.[14] The Argentinian feminist movement was also deeply divided over fundamental issues of sexual ideology and tactics; the most important women's organization, the National Council of Women, rejected the name "feminist" for its philanthropic concerns and could not and would not cooperate with the more radical socialist feminists.[15] In Brazil, according to June Hahner's account, there was less opposition to the demand for the vote for women than in some Latin American countries, but at the same time feminism was tamed and even trivialized: "the pervasive influence of the Roman Catholic church . . . helped to keep the feminist movement within acceptable bounds, preventing feminist attempts to link the oppression of women to motherhood, family, or religion."[16]

Intellectually, women's own participation in eugenics was small. Middle-class women in Brazil, Mexico, and Argentina had broken the barriers to the professions by the 1920s, becoming teachers, lawyers, and civil servants; but the top rungs remained closed to them, and women remained clustered in the lower and less well paid areas of teaching, the bureaucracy, nursing, and pharmacy, much as they did in Europe. Even in Argentina, which had the most advanced system of education in Latin America, the number of women in the professions was small and the difficulties they faced were considerable. Latin American women were therefore not prominent in eugenics circles, except as "auxiliaries" confined largely to the "women's sphere." Women were particularly active as nurses and teachers in the polyclinic and school activities of the Argentine Association of Biotypology, Eugenics, and Social Medicine; this involvement was in keeping with women's educational advances in the country and with their charitable and professional roles, which were organized along gender lines. Men on the whole produced medical science and ran the clinics; women gave comfort and help. Women were therefore not only the objects of eugenics, they were at times its authors, producing eugenics for other women. Mexican eugenics was also distinctive in having five women among the twenty initiating members of the Mexican Eugenics Society; but as

14. Macias, *Against All Odds* [note 13].
15. This account is drawn from Carlson, *¡Feminismo!* [note 13], esp. chaps. 4 and 9.
16. Hahner, *Emancipating the Female Sex* [note 13], p. 154.

the society grew, female membership did not grow correspondingly, a reflection of the limits to professional education for Mexican women and the fundamentally conservative gender ideology inscribed within eugenics.

At the same time, as a region of underdevelopment and gross social inequalities, all the problems connected with sexuality, gender, and motherhood which were associated with eugenics in Europe appeared in exaggerated form in Latin America, thereby providing the political space for a eugenics of puericulture, maternity, and fertility. Working-class women suffered from high maternal death rates and from hard labor in the domestic economy and agriculture, as well as from high levels of participation at very low wages in selective areas of the market economy, such as the textile industry. Infant mortality rates in Brazil and Mexico were extremely high by the standards of the industrialized countries of Europe. Anna Macias comments, "In 1907, with only one-fifth the population of Paris, Mexico City had twice as many *registered* prostitutes, and Paris was supposed to be the sin city of the West. Another sign of dysfunction in Mexican society was that about 30 percent of Mexican mothers were single parents. In addition, about 80 percent of the adult population lived in *amasiato*, or free union, yet illegitimate children had no legal rights to inheritance and could not investigate their paternity."[17] She remarks that while poor women lived in misery, middle-class women had their own though different problems of lack of education, political rights, and legal equality. Everywhere patriarchal values predominated. Antimodernist ideas about women and their roles were widely shared by men on the left and right, even as the actual behavior and experiences of women shattered the familiar myths of gender and family.

This was the context in which a negative eugenics appeared in Latin America. It was a reproductive discourse that made "woman"—notably the poor, laboring, mixed-race woman—the object of a negative eugenics, and in so doing gave her a new eugenic identity. We can think of the concept of the "mothers of the race" and their behaviors—in either "avoiding pregnancy," terminating pregnancy, or "abusing" pregnancy (by vicious or immoral acts)—as being constructed *by* eugenists out of hereditary science to become the key representations that shaped public policy. As a cate-

17. Macias, *Against All Odds* [note 13], p. 13.

gory of historical construction and perception, gender of course includes men; some of the policies of negative eugenics were directed exclusively toward men, thereby constituting the male sex as eugenic beings as well.

A second factor in the emergence of a negative reproductive eugenics in Latin America was its science. It is tempting to think of the meliorism of Lamarckian biology as an inherent feature; since the effects of social reform were expected to be inherited, a negative eugenics of reproduction may have seemed unnecessary. And it is true that many people adopted Lamarkian biology for this reason—because it seemed an optimistic and progressive science. Yet this was not the only way that Lamarckism could be read.[18] A neo-Lamarckian eugenist could equally well argue that the accumulated effects of damaging environments had created a tainted heredity that no amount of social reforms could improve quickly.[19] This view could lead to the pessimistic conclusion that eugenics required some kind of direct control of reproduction. Such an argument was in fact made by a colleague of Pinard, the biologist Frédéric Houssay, in support of both neo-Lamarckism and the enforced sterilization of grossly unfit individuals, such as "chronic alcoholics."[20] There was therefore no contradiction between neo-Lamarckian biology and more extreme policies.

Which reading was made depended on local circumstances and larger ideological factors. In Latin America, the third factor that defined the scope of a negative eugenics was the Roman Catholic church. From the beginning, and alone of the major institutions of the West, the church opposed an extreme reproductive eugenics, for it took human reproduction as a sphere within its own rightful authority and did not cede that authority easily to secular science. Ac-

18. For a discussion of meliorism and Lamarckism (and its limits), see Greta Jones, *Social Darwinism and English Thought* (Sussex: Harvester Press, 1980), pp. 78–87.

19. S. Herbert, "Eugenics and Socialism," *Eugenics Review* 2 (April 1910–January 1911): 116–23, said that Marxists tended to adopt Lamarckism because of their political conviction that economic change could effect radical hereditary change; but he reminded his readers that the German eugenist Wilhelm Schallmeyer had argued that if the effects of the environment were accumulated by inheritance, in successive generations bad effects could cause a group to degenerate. Rejection of Lamarckism and adoption of Mendelism would therefore represent a defense of the working class.

20. Frédéric Houssay, "Eugénique sélection et déterminisme des tares," in *Problems in Eugenics* (London: Eugenics Education Society, 1912), pp. 155–58.

cording to the church, spiritual values in marriage ranked higher than physical ones; the purpose of marriage was reproduction, and the right to reproduce within marriage was therefore unalienable. Moreover, the fruits of reproduction were taken as an expression of God's will; the church therefore did not prohibit the marriages of individuals with hereditary diseases or push out of God's kingdom the physically or mentally "unfit." The church opposed eugenics precisely because it reversed these priorities—because it attacked the rights of individuals within marriage, deformed what it believed was the proper function of sexuality, and perverted the moral sense of the human species. More specifically, the church rejected sterilization as an assault on the integrity of the human body which had no justification in science, morality, or Catholic doctrine.

As the eugenics movement gained ground in western Europe, the Catholic church became alarmed by the zeal to interfere in human reproduction. In 1920 the Catholic National Congress in Britain criticized eugenics as incompatible with Catholic values. In 1924, at one of the first public presentations of eugenics in Italy, the delegates hesitated to express extreme positions on sexuality and reproduction which went against Catholic doctrine.[21] An official ban on eugenics was finally announced in the papal bull of Pius XI in December 1930; called *Casti Connubii* (Of Human Marriage), the encyclical reasserted the church's authority in the sphere of the family, marriage, and sexuality, and prohibited birth control, abortion, sterilization, and eugenics as violations of Catholic principles.[22]

While many eugenists in Latin America denied the legitimacy of the church in the sphere of reproduction, they could not easily dislodge its power to delimit the terms of the debate, even where the church's role was circumscribed by the legal separation of church and state (as it was in Mexico, Uruguay, and Brazil) and where such secular ideas as divorce had been accepted (as in Uruguay in 1905 and Mexico in 1917).[23] Only in the anticlerical and secularized set-

21. Claudio Pogliano, "Scienza e stirpe: Eugenica in Italia (1912–1939)," *Passato e Presente* 5 (1984): 61–97.

22. The church's stand on eugenics and reproduction did not prevent the church in Germany from signing a concordat with the Nazis in 1938. The church also had little to say about eugenics and racism, and only weakly protested the racial persecution of the Jews under fascism. This issue is discussed further in Chapter 5.

23. Because many eugenists approached the human body and sexuality in secular and rationalistic terms, they wanted to see a real separation of church and state, and

ting of Mexico, and then only briefly and in one state, was eugenic sterilization accepted. This does not mean that eugenic sterilization had no Latin American advocates. A social policy that was considered scientifically reasonable, modern, rational, and forward-looking as a medical and public-health measure in Europe seemed all those things to people used to looking to Europe for their scientific and cultural ideas. Psychiatrists and physicians in legal medicine and mental hygiene were especially prone to suggest involuntary sterilization for "gross degenerates." At the First Brazilian Eugenics Congress in Brazil in 1929, for example, Levi Carneiro publicly defended sterilization.[24] According to Ernani Lopes, president of the League of Mental Hygiene, a Dr. Alvaro Ramos had already gone ahead and carried out eugenic sterilizations on women diagnosed as exhibiting sexual derangement and "perversity syndrome."[25]

More often, *public* proposals for sterilization produced an outcry against "brutal zootechnics."[26] In Argentina, a survey of medical doctors in the 1930s showed that only two openly declared themselves to be in favor of obligatory measures.[27] Victor Delfino, who much admired the U.S. sterilization laws, said such laws would be ferociously resisted in his country because of "gross prejudice," something he regretted because it prevented eugenics from aiding the working classes, who in his view most needed "rigorous" policies.[28] The Spanish socialist and jurist Luis Jiménez de Asúa, who

the development of a civil eugenics in place of a Catholic eugenics; this was the thesis of Enrique Díaz de Guijarro, in "La eugenesia y la reciente legislación del matrimonio en América Latina," *Crónica Médica* 61 (1944): 230–36, 282–95.

24. Amanda Rossi Aninat, *Eugenesia y su legislación* (Santiago: Nacimiento, 1941), p. 256.

25. Ernani Lopes, in *Archivos Brasileiros de Hygiene Mental* 4(3) (1931): 247. This makes one think that eugenic sterilizations, perhaps disguised as purely medical procedures, were more common in mental and correctional institutions than is realized. Other proposals for sterilization are Alberto Farani, "Como evitar os proles degenerados," *Archivos Brasileiros de Hygiene Mental* 4(3) (1931): 169–79; and Cunha Lopes, *Da esterilização em psiquiatria* (Rio de Janerio: Separada dos Archivos Brasileiros de Neuratria e Psiquiatria, 1934), p. 10. Cunha Lopes praised the new German sterilization law as a "gigantic advance"; this turn toward a more extreme eugenics in the 1930s is discussed in Chapters 5 and 6.

26. Juan Santos Fernández, "La eugenesia en Buenos Aires," *Semana Médica* (July 10, 1919): 41–43.

27. Carlos Bernaldo de Quirós, *Delincuencia venérea (estudio eugénico jurídico)* (Buenos Aires: n.p., 1934), p. 167.

28. Victor Delfino, "La eugénica en los Estados Unidos," *Semana Médica* (October 2, 1919): 403–4.

lectured extensively on law and eugenics in Latin America in the 1920s and 1930s and who eventually settled in Argentina in 1939, also said that Catholicism, rather than scientific doubt, was the single most important factor inhibiting the development of a more radical eugenics in the region.[29]

"Matrimonial Eugenics": The Italian-Argentine Connection

A negative reproductive eugenics nonetheless developed in Latin America within the parameters of religious proscription, sexual and gender ideology, and scientific outlooks. It was most clearly articulated in the 1930s in the Argentine Association of Biotypology, Eugenics, and Social Medicine, at a moment of perceived crisis in the nation. The association's Italian connection is another interesting dimension to the story; it sheds light on a fascist variant of Latin eugenics, on which very little has been written.

As we saw in Chapter 2, the large number of Italians in Argentina (43 percent of the more than three million immigrants who settled in the country between 1880 and 1930) set the context for close cultural and scientific contacts between the two countries. The Argentine association, which opened its doors in 1932, was modeled on the Institute of Biotypology founded by a physician, Nicola Pende, in Genoa in the 1920s. The fact that its eugenics was based on a strange Italian hereditarian-typological science reminds us once again that twentieth-century eugenics had many scientific and social sources, not one. Pende's "biotypology" was only one of a number of human classificatory sciences that developed in Europe and Latin America in the 1920s and 1930s. Showing many continuities with older classificatory schemes in anthropology and criminology, such as Cesare Lombroso's scheme for distinguishing criminal types according to their physiognomy and craniometry, biotypology was more sophisticated in its scientific base yet fundamentally similar in its idealization and intuitive "sense" of the reality of the types. The

---

29. Luis Jiménez de Asúa, *Libertad de amor y derecho a morir: Ensayos de un criminalista sobre eugenesia y eutanasia* (Buenos Aires: Losado, 1942), p. 39. For a review of Latin American views of eugenic legislation, see Aninat, *Eugenesia y su legislación* [note 24], pp. 138–56.

idea of the "biotype" was intrinsically imprecise, since human populations are infinitely variable and all attempts to divide them categorically into fixed groups, whether racial or "constitutional," are doomed to be arbitrary and controversial. Biotypological science was therefore a means for projecting racial identities onto individuals and groups and drawing invidious distinctions between them. As racism intensified in Europe as well as in Latin America in the 1930s, biotypology found many advocates.[30] In France a biotypological society was founded in 1932, with its own scientific journal; Corrado Gini took biotypology and eugenics as his theme at the Latin International Federation's congress held in Paris in 1937. In Latin America, books on biotypology, especially in relation to hereditary disease and crime, continued to be popular well into the 1940s.[31]

Pende's goal was to use his science to identify and measure the six fundamental, constitutional biotypes that he believed made up all human populations. Although the biotypes did not exactly overlap with races, there was an easy slippage from the language of the type to the language of race. Individuals were assigned to their type by detailed anatomical and physiological analysis, in which endocrinology played a large part. While the basic features of the type were believed to follow Mendelian patterns of inheritance, each individual's heredity was also presumed to be open to degenerative environmental factors. In this way, a place was kept in heredity theory for blastophthoric influences on the germ plasm; alcohol, tobacco, drugs, and venereal diseases were viewed as not only bad in themselves but bad for the offspring, causing lasting hereditary effects on the population. Eugenic regulation and improvement of the biotypes of the nation were believed to be possible through the control

30. See Davydd J. Greenwood, *The Taming of Evolution: The Persistence of Nonevolutionary Views in the Study of Humans* (Ithaca: Cornell University Press, 1984), for a general analysis of various biotypological and constitutional schema. Corrado Gini, in his talk to the International Latin Federation of Eugenics in 1937, said the biotype should be thought of as a mental rather than a statistical category and that therefore in a sense it was arbitrary. See Gini, "Biotypologie et eugénique," in Fédération Internationale Latine des Sociétés d'Eugénique, I Congrès Latin d'Eugénique, *Rapport* (Paris: Masson, 1937), p. 203.

31. An interesting late convert was the leader of the Mexican eugenics movement, Dr. Alfredo Saavedra; see his *Una lección de trabajo social* (Mexico City: n.p., n.d.), which devoted a long chapter to biotypology as an "integral" science of work and social problems. The book was probably written in the 1950s.

of blastophthoric influences.[32] Biotypology also intertwined with Freudian, Adlerian, and other psychological approaches to mental health, a connection that gave psychotherapy in general a peculiarly hereditarian and at times endocrinological orientation.[33]

The main purpose of biotypology was to ensure a knowledge and efficient development of the biotypes in the nation, since each biotype was believed to show distinctive functional aptitudes, psychic pathologies, and susceptibilities to illness and crime. Registering and treating the biotypes, it was argued, would make for better breeding and a stronger, more efficient nation. Correct identification of the biotype would allow medical scientists to allocate human beings to their proper places in the nation's biopolitical economy. Another key word was "orthogenetics," meaning the scientific correction of departures from biotypological norms. In the Genoa school, for instance, Pende had established a special house for children who presented "anomalies" of a moral kind and, according to the biotypologist, required a kind of preventive detention. Pende considered the study and inventory of biotypes to be essential to the fascist state, because it provided Mussolini with a scientific profile of the nation's health, fertility, and identity.[34]

Pende's visit to Buenos Aires in 1930 came at a critical moment in Argentina's history. The military coup of that year brought to a close a decade or more of the progressive incorporation of new immigrant groups into political life and the development of new intellectual and cultural activities. The coup was followed by a long period of antiegalitarian politics, corrupt elections, and the emergence of nationalist ideologies of various kinds. The search for organic, statist solutions to heterogeneity in social life which would transcend class conflicts was a common feature of many of the conservative formulations that developed in the period.

32. See, for instance, the link between Mendelian and essentially pre-Mendelian language in Arturo R. Rossi's "Curso sintético de medicina constitucional y biotypología: Herencia y constitución," *ABEMS* 1 (May, 1 1933): 12–14, where he referred to the laws of Mendel, the laws of Galton, the laws of eugenics, and blastophthoria as all part of his science. Eight years later, in "Herencia, constitución, eugenesia y ortogénesis," *ABEMS* 95 (February–March 1941): 1–24, it is the language of Morgan, biometrics, and Mendelism that is combined with blastophthoria.

33. For an interesting analysis of a similar intertwining of ideas in Spain, see Thomas F. Glick, "Psicoanálisis, reforma sexual y política en la España de entreguerras," *Estudios de Historia Social* 16–17 (1981): 7–25.

34. Pende dedicated his book *Bonifaca umana razionale e biologia politica* (Bologna: Capelli, 1933) to Mussolini.

Pende's visit stimulated a diverse group of obstetricians, puericulturists, demographers, criminologists, and medical legal theorists who had long been preoccupied with the woes of modernity—alcoholism, tuberculosis, prostitution, illegitimacy, low natality, and high rates of infant mortality—to create a new organization to tackle the medical aspects of the social crisis. The Association of Biotypology's large membership, its technical commissions, its training school, its scientific journal, and its polyclinic, where segments of the population were assessed and treated, gave eugenics new visibility in the capital city.

Argentina in 1932 was not a fascist state, but the institutional success of the association owed a lot to its resonance with authoritarian political and intellectual currents at that time. The worldwide depression further exacerbated social problems by causing high rates of unemployment, poverty, and ill health. In addition to the huge fall in export earnings, the depression caused a reassessment of immigration as a valid source of population. With the reduction of immigration and a growing disillusionment as to its "racial quality," doctors turned their eyes on the population *in* Argentina to see how it might be given a coherent identity and strength.[35]

The activities of the association centered on a cluster of themes: demography, fertility and natality, immigration, and heredity. Cutting across and uniting many of them was the issue of gender and reproduction. Pende had developed his science within a fascist society in which the church had kept its privileged position (in the concordat between the church and the fascist state in 1929). Furthermore, as Lesley Caldwell has shown, in fascist Italy the "repertoires of meaning" of women as mothers within the sacred institution of marriage were well established.[36] Italy was pronatalist, and the demographic theme and the "difesa della stirpe" (defense of the stock) were part of Mussolini's rhetoric from the early stages of the Fascist regime; but they were developed more consistently in the 1930s, when they became available as ideologies and social practices for emulation and selective appropriation by the Argentine Association of Biotypology.

In the summer of 1933, the vice president of the association, Oc-

---

35. See remarks about Argentine eugenics printed in the Mexican eugenics journal *Boletín de la Sociedad Eugénica Mexicana* 1 (October 25, 1932): 1–2.

36. Lesley Caldwell, "Reproducers of the Nation: Women and the Family in Fascist Policy," in *Rethinking Italian Fascism*, ed. David Forgacs (London: Lawrence & Wishart, 1986), p. 115.

tavio López, traveled to Italy to study biotypology and to discuss eugenics with such religious figures as Father Agostino Gemelli, rector of the Sacred Heart University in Milan and a eugenics advocate who as early as 1924 had played a part in steering Italian eugenists away from the more extreme ideas of the British and Americans.[37] In the wake of the church's condemnation of eugenics, sterilization, abortion, and birth control, a real question existed as to whether and how eugenics could be practiced in Catholic countries. Gemelli argued, however, that the church was not opposed to eugenics per se, only to the use of aggressive force to solve eugenic problems. When eugenics did not violate the "natural laws of motherhood," when it used methods of persuasion to form a eugenic conscience in the home and to prevent "disgraceful" unions (genetically or "racially"), then eugenics was permissible within a Catholic society. López then asked himself and his fellow Argentinians the following question: Was this goal for eugenics really scientific, in its minimum program and its vast social sphere? He answered in the affirmative—that a true "matrimonial" eugenics in its most practical form opened a wide array of investigations and remedies, involving the family and offspring, marriage and work, immigration and migration.[38]

In Argentina the eugenists therefore worked to achieve racial improvement through the measurement of biotypes, matrimonial selection based on the principles of heredity and adaptation, and the orthogenetic correction of individuals who departed from the correct hereditary norms. Biotypology was used to evaluate "ancestral determinants" and the grades of reaction to the environment in deviants. On the sexual side, eugenists proposed sexual education to "subdue the sexual instinct" and turn it to eugenic ends; attacked sexual "delinquency," homosexuality, and sexual license; and offered advice and evaluations on the type of racial unions they believed would be "harmonious" and produce hereditarily healthy offspring. They suggested proscription of marriages between "widely separate races" as causing degenerations that threatened Argentinian nationality.

The most important proposal put forward by the Argentinian eu-

37. Pogliano, in "Scienza e stirpe" [note 21], describes the role of Gemelli at the first important public meetings of the Italian eugenics society in Milan in 1924.
38. Octavio V. López, "Cristianismo y eugenesia," *ABEMS* 1 (August 1, 1933): 6–7.

genists was the biotypological identity card ("ficha biotipológica"), an idea they took from Pende. Pende planned to have free bio-typological dispensaries in every great Italian urban center, similar to the one he actually developed in Genoa.[39] The Argentinian euge-nists of the 1930s imagined the ficha not as a voluntary, personal record of family history but as an obligatory instrument that would permit the state to register and manipulate the population.[40] A vari-ant of the identity card which they favored especially was the school biotypological identity card, an idea that was accepted by the Coun-cil on Education and the Schools Department for the Province of Buenos Aires in 1933. A school and national "log" of biotypes would make possible the creation of a kind of "national identity register," which, biotypologists argued, would aid greatly in the ra-tional management of the biological patrimony of the nation. It would allow doctors to monitor changes in the individual's biotype and carry out medical "orthogenetic" treatment in correctional schools for delinquents.[41] Assessments of children along these lines was in fact the major work of the polyclinic that opened in 1933. The eugenists proposed combining the scheme of national identity cards with a new judicial police, who would enforce a new social security code and create children's courts.[42]

But since it was mainly through women, or more precisely moth-erhood, that the future biotypological identity and health of the na-tion was seen to be produced, the eugenists in the association fo-cused particular attention on the regulation of female biotypes.

39. Julio M. Escobar Saenz, "Biotipología y eugenesia en la organización del esta-do," *ABEMS* 1 (July 15, 1933): 15; and Eugène Schreider, "L'école biotypologique italienne: Tendances et méthodes," *Biotypologie* 1 (March 1933): 64–97. The idea of a medical-eugenic identity card took a variety of forms; in France, Georges Schreiber proposed issuing families a "livret" or record of the genealogy and hereditary history of family members, and the idea was adopted enthusiastically by Renato Kehl in Brazil.

40. The idea was taken up in other Latin American countries; see, for example, the reference to obligatory biotypological cards at the First Peruvian Congress of Eugenics in 1939; cf. Susan Solano's "Cartilla biotipológico obligatorio contribuye a la higiene de la raza," in *Primera Jornada Peruana de Eugenesia* (Lima, 1940), pp. 96–101. The idea of a national inventory of the hereditary value of all the inhabitants of the country was part of Nazi eugenics as well; see Bock, "Racism and Sexism" [note 6].

41. Arturo R. Rossi, "Ficha biotipológica ortogenética escolar," *ABEMS* 1 (July 15, 1933): 12–14. I have no evidence that the school biotypological identity cards were ever actually used.

42. Arturo R. Rossi, "La ficha biotipológica escolar: Sus fundamentos," *ABEMS* 1 (April 1, 1933): 14–16.

Many of the members of the association were puericulturists and obstetricians who had come into eugenics and biotypology through the influence of Pinard, and this puericultarist outlook structured their activities. Pronatalism was another factor in the history of Argentinian eugenics, as it was for many other movements. Pronatalism of course took many forms and had a variety of political meanings.[43] Settlement of the vast Argentinian pampas was a long-standing concern; the notion that "to govern is to populate" was a powerful trope of political discourse and had long helped promote an open immigration policy. But by the 1930s these policies were viewed much more negatively. Many of the immigrants, it was now said, were not of the desired European ancestry, but were of "eastern" or "Oriental" origin (meaning Russian, Syrian, and Lebanese) that made them incommensurable with the "best" of Argentina's racial stock.

As attitudes toward immigration began to change in the late 1920s and early 1930s, then, immigration was no longer seen as an adequate answer to the problems of nationhood and identity; indeed, proposals for immigration restriction became the order of the day. Eugenists turned their attention to the population already in the country and to the adequacy of its reproduction rates and biological vitality. Resort to clandestine abortions, women's work outside the home, the widespread failure to feel an adequate "responsibility" to the nation, "false" democratic values, new sexual customs and the venereal diseases that accompanied them—all were variously blamed for what was presented as a veritable crisis of low fertility of the white population of the country.

All of these problems seemed to converge most especially on women and maternity. The Argentinian biotypologists much admired Mussolini's state rhetoric and programs of "family protec-

43. Before the 1930s, very few countries believed themselves to be suffering from "overpopulation" (the term itself became current then). The causes given for each country's supposed "underpopulation" or "depopulation" varied. They included the negative effects of generalized "degeneration" and modernization, the deaths caused by the Great War (not an issue in Latin America), by civil war (an important issue in Mexico, where the losses of population in the Revolution were enormous), and an initially small population in relation to geographical size (a theme in Brazil and Argentina). Generalized pronatalism had a tendency to become differentiated: most eugenists supposed their own countries to have too many of the "wrong types" of people and too few of the "right types." Eugenists defined the wrong and right types in individual, class, ethnic, and racial terms, depending on the circumstances.

tion," programs whose pronatalist, antiabortion, and antifeminist ideology was highly congruent with their own. The combination of exaltation of maternity and control of sexuality seemed to the Argentinian eugenists a satisfactory answer to the problem of the disintegration of the family by modernity. Eugenics was to be "hogaría y educación maternológica" (the science of the home and the mother); it was to be a rational form of sex education, directed toward subduing the sexual instinct to the eugenic will and toward the remoralization of the family.[44]

Within maternal eugenics, providing child allowances to the poor and reducing health hazards at work took second and third place to stressing the reproductive "obligations of women." The eugenists called for an involuntary state system of surveillance of motherhood and the forcible registration of pregnancy, since pregnancies represented to them the vital germ plasm of the nation. And of course, like so many other eugenists and social reformers, they wrote about the need for compulsory education in the skills of motherhood, which in Argentina was put forward as a female equivalent to compulsory military service for men.[45]

They also advocated using the biotypological identity card to draw up a mandatory "eugenic index of individual value in fertility" ("ficha eugenésica de valuación de fecundad individual"), which would carry information on race, religion, color, and fertility, the latter being measured by a record of pregnancies and childbirth.[46] Pregnant women would be required by law to come under medical care from the third month, so that their health could be monitored, abortion prevented, and correct biotypological and eugenic development achieved. In this way the eugenic-medical supervision of the germ plasm of the nation could be made into a political principle of national strength. Eugenists made clear that women would become the object of eugenic care not as women per se but only as mothers.[47]

44. Carlos Bernaldo de Quirós and Mercedes Rodrigues de Ginocchio, "Educación sexual eugénico maternológica," *Eugenesia* new ser. 3 (February 8, 1942): 7–18.
45. Josué A. Beruti and María de Zurano, "Contribución al estudio del problema de la protección maternal en nuestro país," *ABEMS* 2 (November 1, 1934): 4–6.
46. Josué A. Beruti, Arturo R. Rossi, and María G. Zurano, "Ficha eugénica de valuación de fecundad individual," *ABEMS* 2 (October 1, 1934): 15–16.
47. Beruti drew attention to the radical programs for women as future mothers in Germany and the Nazis' idea of "education for motherhood," which he said could serve as a model for other countries; see ibid. See also C. Bernaldo de Quirós, *Problemas*

Thus it was not the health of the individual woman that mattered but her health in relation to her child, that is, to the future germ plasm of the nation.

The Prenuptial Certificate

Many of the suggestions for negative reproductive eugenics put forward in Latin America operated as a set of prescriptions, creating norms and cultural images that influenced the metaphors used to describe health and the behaviors of the middle and lower classes. Negative eugenics made women's fertility seem a crucial resource of the nation, thus locking women into reproductive roles. It supported racist ideas by proposing that maintaining distance between various ethnic and racial groups was necessary for the prosperity of the nation.

The other plank in the negative eugenics of reproduction, the prenuptial test or certificate for marriage, was a more direct form of eugenic proscription, resulting in some countries in legally binding rules of a negative kind. Many Latin Americans viewed such tests as defining the special form of negative eugenics in Catholic countries, because they acted as direct restraints on unfit unions without entailing the use of surgical or other unacceptable methods.[48] Of all the steps that could have been taken toward the eugenic normalization of the human fabric, this kind of control of birth without birth control went a long way toward giving concrete and practical form to the negative eugenics special to Latin American countries.

There was nothing new in the West about obligatory medical (as opposed to religious) requirements or restrictions on marriage; they had been written into Danish law as early as 1798, for instance, with

---

demográphicos argentina (Buenos Aires: Cruz del Sur, 1942), p. 99, about the need for a "state birth policy" based on the woman as mother.

48. F. Imantoff, "La développement de la médicine préventive en Belgique," ABEMS 2 (December 1, 1934): 14–17, described how, when the Belgian Society of Eugenics (Societé Belge d'Eugénique) had fallen into lethargy and lost membership, it decided to move in a new direction; it renamed itself the Belgian Society of Preventive Medicine and Eugenics and launched a campaign in favor of prenuptial certificates. This move led to a huge increase in interest—the society held 33 meetings on the subject in 1929, 84 in 1930, and 165 in 1931.

little effect. Such examinations had many defenders in the early twentieth century, from feminists concerned with protecting women from venereal infections in marriage to physicians who wished to protect children from the effects of parental infections.[49] In Latin America (and in some countries in Europe), advocacy of prenuptial tests of various kinds had crystallized as eugenic measures in the 1920s and 1930s. They were defended as instruments of race improvement, even though they raised extremely difficult moral issues as well as practical ones of application. Discussion of such tests generated a minispecialty. Many of the people involved were lawyers by training, and they produced a new kind of literature which is now largely unread but which offers the historian of eugenics a fascinating view of a hidden field of comparative marital eugenics.[50] These writers debated whether the tests should be medical or merely juridical (that is, involve medical tests or merely legally binding statements of fitness on the part of the marriage partners); should require medical certificates as well as medical tests; should be voluntary or involuntary; and should apply equally to both sexes or not.

Calls for a ban on the marriages of the unfit were first heard in Latin America in the 1880s and 1890s; they intensified over time as the emphasis on hereditary unfitness increased. In 1910, for instance, the Mexican pamphlet on eugenics by Dr. Fortuno Hernández, called *Hygiene of the Species: Brief Considerations Concerning Human Stirpiculture*, rejected the methods of the "farmyard" but recom-

49. Prenuptial examinations or tests for marriage, on eugenic grounds, were common in many of the states of the United States and in Germany. According to Peter Weingart, in "The Rationalization of Sexual Behavior: The Institutionalization of Eugenics in Germany," *Journal of the History of Biology* 20 (1987): 159–93, there were some 200 counseling centers for prospective couples in Prussia alone by 1931. Compulsory premarital testing for marriage did not become law until the 1935 Nazi Law for the Protection of the Genetic Health of the German People, which also prohibited marriages between Aryans and Jews.

50. E.g., Enrique Díaz de Guijarro, *El examen médico en el seguro de la vida, sus efectos jurídicos* (Buenos Aires: Antología Jurídica, 1941); Carlos Bernaldo de Quirós, *Eugenesia jurídica y social (derecho eugenésico argentino)* (Buenos Aires: Editorial Ideas, 1943); Luis Jiménez de Asúa, *Cuestiones legales de eugenesia, filosofía y política* (Cochabamba, Bolivia: Imprenta Universitaria, 1943); Frías, *El matrimonio* [note 3]; Aninat, *Eugenesia y su legislación* [note 4]; and from Brazil, Teodolino Castiglione, *A eugenia no direito da família* (São Paulo: Saraiva, 1924). Courses in eugenic legislation were also introduced; see, e.g., Enrique Díaz de Guijarro, "La enseñanza de la eugenesia en universidades argentinas," *Crónica Médica* 61 (1944): 151–61, 181–88.

124 · "The Hour of Eugenics"

mended some kind of barrier to the marriages of people with venereal disease, tuberculosis, or alcoholism.[51] In Brazil, Renato Kehl introduced the subject in 1918 at the first meeting of the newly founded São Paulo Eugenics Society.[52] In 1922, at the Sixth Latin
American Medical Congress, the prenuptial certificate was defended
as a solution to depopulation and racial health, and was one of the
motivating factors behind the decision to set up a Pan American
Office of Eugenics (voted into being in 1923). Thereafter the Pan
American meetings on child health and on eugenics constantly called
for the legalization of prenuptial tests. The Latin Americans found
support for their view in the eugenics societies of Belgium and
France, the former holding a conference in 1926 expressly to popularize the idea and endorsing a prenuptial examination as a voluntary
and prudential aid to marriage, not as an obligatory impediment to
it.[53]

Eugenists argued the need for such examinations by pointing to
the hereditary damage that could be eliminated from populations if
the syphilitic or otherwise eugenically unsound individual were
barred from marrying. Since many Latin American countries recognized civil marriage, the eugenists could turn to civil law as a way of
introducing tests and certificates. The neo-Lamarckian orientation of
many eugenists encouraged them to include in their list of banned
conditions a motley collection of contagions and infections. Banning
people with venereal disease from marriage was, for instance, invariably tied up with eugenic terminology. Believing, as so many of
eugenists did, that alcohol could permanently damage the germ
plasm and therefore the next generation, restraint on marriage of the
alcoholic was another common aspect of prenuptial legislation.

The main disagreements among the eugenists revolved around
whether such tests should be voluntary or obligatory. In many parts
of Latin America marriage rates were very low and illegitimacy rates
extremely high. Requiring prenuptial tests and/or certificates as a
method of preventing reproduction by the "unfit" was therefore
patently absurd; the middle class found convenient ways of buying
such certificates, while the poor, with whom the eugenists were

51. Fortuno Hernández, *Higiene de la especie: Breves consideraciones sobre la stir-
picultura humana* (Mexico City: Bouligny y Schmidt, 1910), p. 66.
52. *Annães de eugenia* (São Paulo: Revista do Brasil, 1919), pp. 3–7.
53. Frías, *El matrimonio* [note 3], p. 189.

most concerned, were only put off further from regularizing their unions.[54] Prenuptial tests therefore ran the risk of actually encouraging "immorality," rather than encouraging eugenic practices. Many physicians consequently saw prenuptial examinations as voluntary aids in the encouragement of large and healthy families. This was the position taken by Jorge Frías in his much-cited study of matrimony and eugenics, and some people considered it to be the truly Catholic position on the subject.

Other eugenists pushed to have prenuptial medical tests and certificates introduced as obligatory, state-controlled restraints on "diseased" marriages, along the lines of legislation requiring the Wassermann test for syphilis in the United States.[55] Throughout the 1920s, the matter was much debated by eugenists and medical doctors concerned more broadly with human sanitation and the need to control social diseases. A broad range of diseases and conditions was believed to warrant a prohibition on the right to marriage and the physicians' showed great confidence in urging state intervention in private lives. Syphilis, alcoholism, drug addiction, mental illness, mental deficiency, and even chronic contagious diseases were all considered grounds for excluding individuals from legal forms of reproduction because they were believed to cause immediate infections *and* might produce more permanent hereditary damage to the human species.

These proposals had political effects. By 1928, premarital medical examinations had been mandated by law in Mexico, and marriage licenses were banned in theory for all individuals with chronic and contagious illnesses and for those with conditions transmissible by heredity, as well as those with vices that could endanger the heredity of offspring.[56] The list of conditions and diseases included "mor-

54. The physician Paz Soldán said as much at the Pan American Congress of Eugenics in 1934; by then an involuntary premarital certificate had supposedly been required in Peru for some years, but certificates could so easily be falsified as to render the law farcical. Nevertheless, at the First Peruvian Conference of Eugenics, held in Lima in 1939, the delegates once again voted in favor of obligatory medical certificates for marriage. See the conference report published in *Primera Jornada Peruana de Eugenesia* (Lima, 1940), p. 21. The delegates also voted in favor of annulment of marriages contracted during chronic illnesses and of divorce if one partner acquired chronic, contagious, or hereditary illness during the marriage.

55. Kevles, *In the Name of Eugenics* [note 12], pp. 99–100.

56. Díaz de Guijarro, "La eugenesia y la reciente legislación" [note 23], pp. 283–84.

phine addiction" or dependency on other narcotics, habitual alcoholism, idiocy, and mental illness. In Chile the radical Popular Front proposed more restricted legislation to control venereal disease; the then director of public health, Dr. Salvador Allende, suggested such a bill in Congress in 1939.[57]

In Brazil in 1927, the congressman Amaury de Medeiros presented to the commission on public health in the Federal Congress a bill calling for voluntary prenuptial examinations, which he described as a form of "constructive" (as opposed to negative) eugenics compatible with "Brazilian traditions."[58] People with grave physical defects and transmissible diseases were to be examined. Many congressmen opposed the plan, but Medeiros had the support of the eugenists Kehl, Penna, Peixoto, and others on sanitary grounds, though Kehl, for one, hoped to see the examinations made obligatory. Medeiros's death that same year stopped further legislative action. In the 1930s, however, worries about the entry of poor European immigrants into the already strained Brazilian economy caused nationalist and antiforeign sentiment to intensify and support for eugenic legislation to grow. The eugenists actively pressed their views during the debates of the constituent assembly that was elected after the coup of 1930.[59] Their success in introducing eugenic measures at the national level is a sign of how far eugenics had penetrated as a language of interpretation of the national condition.

First, the eugenists' proposal to make the "promotion of eugenic education" a responsibility of the national state was written into Brazil's new constitution of 1934.[60] Given the high rate of illiteracy in Brazil (probably 80 percent) and the inadequate system of primary or secondary education, we must read "eugenic education" as signif-

57. Elsa Wigold Aguirre, "El certificado médico prenupcial" (thesis, Universidad de Chile, 1945), p. 58. The termination of the Popular Front prevented passage of the bill.

58. His original proposal was reprinted after his death; see Amaury de Medeiros, "O exame prenupcial," *Archivos do Instituto Medico-Legal e do Gabinete de Identificação* 2 (November 1931): 71–86.

59. A discussion of these efforts is provided by Teodolino Castiglione, *A eugenia no direito da famila: O codigo civil brasileiro e a lei sobre a organização e proteção da familia perante a eugenia* (São Paulo: Saraiva, 1942), esp. pp. 14–19. The new Ministry of Labor, created in 1934 under Vargas, was one place where eugenical matters were discussed.

60. Renato Kehl, *Lições de eugenia* (Rio de Janeiro: Editora Brasil, 1935), pp. 235–43.

icant for the symbolic importance the national state attached to "race improvement" in the 1930s. Second, as the Catholic church grew closer to the Brazilian state in the 1930s, winning such important constitutional concessions as the legality of church marriages and the prohibition of divorce, eugenists found the ideological environment unpropitious for programs of state-sanctioned sterilization which some eugenists—including Kehl, Oscar Fontanelle, and Renato Pacheco Silva—had proposed for the "grossly degenerate unfit."[61] Also thwarted were efforts by eugenists, or by radical workers and doctors on the other side of the political spectrum, to legalize birth control, or abortion in exceptional cases, for eugenic, feminist, or sanitary reasons.[62] On the other hand, the eugenists and their allies were successful in introducing a "nubente" clause requiring prospective marital couples to present medical proof of their mental and physical health before marriage, a requirement written into the constitution eight years before its equivalent in France, under the Vichy regime. The prenuptial examination was obligatory; but the law was qualified by the statement that its application would take into consideration the regional conditions of the country (a recognition of the absence of any administrative apparatus that could oversee the application of the law, and indeed the absence of adequate numbers of health officials anywhere but in the larger cities).[63] Nonetheless, the fact that eugenics was made part of the national constitution of Brazil indicates the privileged place of science as a discourse in modern Brazil and the weight attached to "race improvement" in the national state.

The Brazilian prenuptial law applied, theoretically, to both sexes. In other countries, the laws were directed specifically toward men, reflecting the differential constructions of gender within eugenics. Women, as we have seen, were constituted within eugenics as reproductive-maternal beings. Men, on the other hand, were seen as essentially sexual beings. Lower-class men especially were thought to be sexually irresponsible and likely to be infected with disease.

61. Ibid., p. 225.
62. Ibid., pp. 212–17.
63. Since a very large number of unions in Brazil were extralegal (over 50 percent in many regions), the effectiveness of the law was doubtful. Whether the law, strictly speaking, deserved the name "eugenic" was also a moot point; to Mendelians it did not, since it was meant to screen primarily for venereal infections, which Mendelians believed had no long-term hereditary effects.

Prenuptial tests were therefore put forward as particularly necessary for men, as a means of preventing their licentiousness and infections from harming women and thereby the hereditary health of the nation. In Argentina, for example, the prenuptial law (law 12,331) passed in 1937 instituted obligatory examination, registration, and treatment of venereal disease. The law was based on straightforward medical criteria and on the neo-Lamarckian assumption that venereal infections could have hereditary and therefore racial effects. It applied, however, only to men.[64]

Mexico and Negative Eugenics

Mexico was one Latin American nation that experimented with eugenic sterilization. Although the experiment was extremely short-lived, it provides an interesting exception to the rule that, as an Italian claimed, "the Latin mentality rejects sterilization."[65] It also is instructive about the politics of negative eugenics in Latin America.

The meaning of the Mexican Revolution—for politics, for social life, for nationalism—is continually being reassessed. The upheavals encompassed a variety of revolutions—a local peasant revolution concerned primarily with land reform, for instance, and a national revolution concerned with industrialization, the creation of a middle class, and the formation of a strong state bureaucracy. Although the country was, like the rest of Latin America, overwhelmingly Catholic, the official ideology of the revolution was anticlerical and materialist. Early in the revolution, complete separation between church and state was reiterated as a fundamental principle of the Mexican Republic. Divorce was legalized and the secularization of primary education advanced as a way to curb the power of the church. The country was in a state of civil war between 1910 and 1920, and it was not until 1926 that the laws regulating church power were put into effect, a move that led to determined resistance by church authorities and by much of the traditional middle class. In many states of the republic, especially the more radically anticlerical states of Jalisco and Veracruz, this resistance led to armed revolt, in which

64. On Argentina, see Roberto Mac-Lean y Estenos, *La eugenesia en América*, (Mexico City: Instituto de Investigaciones Sociales, Cuadernos de Sociología, Imprenta Universitaria, 1952), pp. 37–38, on law 12,331.

65. Uriel Sperapini, in "La sterilizzazione eugenica," *ABEMS* 3 (June 1, 1936): 6.

peasants joined the side of the church. After 1929, religious education was once again tolerated, but church-state relations continued to be fraught with tension.[66] By 1935, anticlericism had in fact reduced the total number of priests to fewer than five hundred in all of Mexico. Says J. Lloyd Mecham, "In half of the states, no priests were allowed to function at all, although the practice of religion was guaranteed by the Constitution."[67] Despite the onslaught on its prerogatives, however, the church retained considerable ideological power in Mexico, and the authority of Catholicism in its traditional spheres of the family, marriage, and gender generally remained great. The depth of the resistance to secularism points to the gulf that often separated the people in power at the national and state levels from ordinary Mexicans.

Thus when eugenics was put forward as a radical solution to the problems of racial health and nationality—radical in that it dealt with the highly sensitive topics of marriage, gender, sexuality, and sexual disease in a fundamentally non-Catholic, rationalistic, and materialist fashion—it was viewed as a further and dreadful assault on Catholic and traditional values. In the circumstances, a negative and extreme eugenics could be introduced only as part of a revolutionary program of public health and in a situation in which the authorities believed they had some control over public opinion. This interpretation is borne out by the history of the sex-education campaign and of sexual sterilization.

The Mexican Society of Eugenics had emerged in 1932 in a period of conservative consolidation of the state and growing political nationalism. It had good contacts with the federal and state health authorities and cannot be considered to have been completely out of sympathy with the goals of the national state.[68] Its members can

66. Jean Meyer writes that the church in this period operated as a kind of substitute opposition to the revolution; see his "Mexico: Revolution and Reconstruction in the 1920s," in *The Cambridge History of Latin America*, ed. Leslie Bethell (Cambridge: Cambridge University Press, 1986), 5: 155–94.

67. J. Lloyd Mecham, *Church and State in Latin America: A History of Politico-Ecclesiastical Relations* (Chapel Hill: University of North Carolina Press, 1966), pp. 404–5.

68. *Boletín de la Sociedad Eugénica Mexicana* 6 (September 21, 1932): 1–4 describes the several hundred official notices sent to federal and state authorities in the first few months of the society's existence. The society had representatives from twelve Mexican states. The *Boletín* changed its name to *Eugenesia* with no. 19, December 31, 1932.

probably be fairly classified as secular and materialist in outlook, many of them speaking out on the need for sex education and even eugenic sterilization if the Mexican "race" were to be improved. Like most of their Latin colleagues, the Mexican eugenists combined modernist with antimodernist attitudes—they were pronatalist and antifeminist, anticinema, antialcohol, and antipornography. Several of them also promoted birth control as a remedy for Mexico's "underpopulation," on the grounds that the rational control of unwanted births would ensure that children born to the poor would be adequately supported and in good health.[69]

Sex education was a particular concern of eugenists, as it was for many radicals in Mexico, as a way of disciplining the sex instinct and subduing it to "rational" goals.[70] Often called for and almost never implemented, sex education was one of the lost causes of Latin American eugenics.[71] In Mexico, numerous efforts had been made to discuss sex education, to publicize its function in healthy marriages, to teach it to doctors and teachers. Things came to a head in July 1932, when the National Block of Revolutionary Women in Mexico City petitioned the secretary of public education for the introduction of sex education in technical schools and suggested that the Mexican Eugenics Society be asked to draw up a plan of action. At the secretary's request, the society put forward the "Project for Sex Education and the Prophylaxis of Venereal Diseases and Alcoholism," in which it recommended sex education for all children under the age of sixteen in state schools. The recommendation led to a storm of protest in the medical and national press. The society never quite lived down the scandal, and in 1934 the secretary of education was forced to resign.[72]

The eugenists were equally radical on the matter of sterilization.

69. For eugenic demands for birth control, see Angel Brioso Vasconcelos, "La esterilización eugénica," Boletín de la Sociedad Eugénica Mexicana 18 (December 17, 1932): 1–2.

70. Many feminists supported sex education and coeducation, easy divorce, and legalization of birth control, as well as campaigns against drugs, alcohol, and prostitution. See Macias, Against All Odds [note 13], passim.

71. Sex education was also part of eugenics movements in Europe and Britain; see, e.g., R. A. Lowe, "Eugenists, Doctors, and the Quest for National Efficiency: An Educational Crusade, 1900–1939," History of Education 8(4) (1979): 293–306.

72. See Alfredo Saavedra M., México en la educación sexual (de 1860 a 1959) (Mexico City: B. Costa-Amic, 1967), pp. 31–101. This account of the controversies over sex education in Mexico is by the leader of the eugenics movement in the country.

In 1921 Dr. Felix Palaviccini, the organizer and president of the first national conference on the child, proposed eugenic sterilization of criminals; the proposal was narrowly approved by seven votes.[73] In the 1930s, when the eugenics movement became organized, the Mexican Eugenics Society had apparently much closer connections to U.S. scientists than did the societies in countries farther south, such as Brazil and Argentina, and several of the Mexican members took the line that since eugenic sterilization was viewed favorably in the "vanguard" countries—the United States, Sweden, Norway, and elsewhere—Mexico should take a positive stand toward it also.[74]

Events almost overtook the society when on July 6, 1932, shortly after the society came into being, the fanatically anticlerical governor of Veracruz, Adalberto Tejeda, authorized the first and only eugenic sterilization law in the country. Tejeda was one of the last of the autonomous caudillos of the revolutionary movement. His support came from people in favor of agrarian reform; he was opposed, often strenuously, by the elite of Veracruz and by the traditional middle class there and elsewhere.[75] Eugenic sterilization, then, can be understood as an expression of radical anticlericalism and secularism and of the hope that the successes of science in improving livestock could be brought to bear on human beings.[76]

The eugenic law of Veracruz was drawn up by a sociologist and economist, Salvador Mendoza, with the advice of the Mexican Eugenics Society. By the new law, eugenic sterilization was to become

73. According to M. T. Nisot, *La question eugénique dans les divers pays* (Brussels: Faile, 1927), p. 357, other biologists and social scientists had envisaged the sterilization of criminals and degenerates (i.e., punitive as well as medical sterilization).

74. See, e.g., Brioso Vasconcelos, "Esterilización eugénica" [note 69], pp. 1–2.

75. Romana Falcón and Soledad García, *La semilla en el surco: Adalberto Tejeda y el radicalismo en Veracruz, 1883–1960* (Mexico City: Colegio de México and Gobierno del Estado de Veracruz, 1986).

76. Ibid., pp. 269–70. Another factor that played an indirect part in the search for human improvement via eugenic laws was the Depression, which in addition to causing increased hardship in Mexico cut off the safety valve of emigration to the United States.

The question whether eugenics could be a project of the left is disputed by historians. Michael Freeden, "Eugenics and Progressive Thought: A Study of Ideological Affinity," *Historical Journal* 22 (1979): 645–71, points to the ideological similarity between progressive outlooks and eugenics. Greta Jones takes the opposite view, that eugenics was inherently reactionary; see her "Eugenics and Social Policy between the Wars," *Historical Journal* 25 (1982): 717–28. Diane Paul discusses left-wing ideas of state-imposed eugenics in "Eugenics and the Left," *Journal of the History of Ideas* 45 (1984): 567–90.

one aspect of a new service within the state department of health, to be known as the Section on Eugenics and Mental Hygiene. The service was to focus on inheritance, criminality, prostitution, alcoholism, and the mental condition of children. The law also introduced sex education in the schools, made the registration and treatment of venereal infections obligatory, legalized birth control, abolished many small bars and taverns, and restricted the sale of alcohol elsewhere. According to a commentary on the law, birth control was legalized because the middle and "desirable" classes were resorting to contraception and therefore were not reproducing, while the lower, "less desirable" classes reproduced to excess, causing a degeneration in the Mexican race. The new law, it was claimed, would put birth control in reach of everyone, with positive results for eugenic improvement.[77]

Finally, the law also legalized eugenic sterilization in "clear cases of idiocy" and for the "degenerate mad," the "incurably ill," and "delinquents." Safeguards against abuse of the law would be provided by requiring "the agreement of three competent physicians that eugenic legislation in the particular case was necessary." Sterilization would be directed toward "controlling genetic incapacity" and preserving sexual function (a reference to the fact that the law involved surgical sterilization and not castration, a distinction not everyone understood).

A few months after the passage of the sterilization law, Tejeda's term (his second) as governor of his native state came to an end in a moment of violent conflict between radicals and conservatives and an intense campaign to disarm the resisting *campesinos*. In the circumstances, it is highly unlikely that actual sterilizations took place. In 1942, at a meeting of the Mexican Eugenics Society (by then a much smaller organization), the Mexican biologist José Rulfo reviewed the impact of eugenic legislation around the world and raised a question specifically about the fate of the legislation in Veracruz. It is clear that he had no information about it.[78] Moreover,

77. The law itself was announced in *Boletín de la Sociedad Eugénica Mexicana* 2 (August 25, 1932): 4; the law was printed, with commentary, in "Ley de eugenesia e higiene mental de Veracruz," *Eugenesia* 23 (March 10, 1933): 3–6. Commentary is also found in "Consideraciones a la ley número 352 del Estado de Veracruz," by Dr. Augustín Hernández Mejia, in *Boletín de la Sociedad Eugénica Mexicana* 12 (November 4, 1932): 2–3.

78. José Rulfo, "Ponencia de eugenesia," *Eugenesia* new ser. 3 (May 1942): 3–26.

no sooner had the law been passed in Veracruz than many eugenists began to express their doubts about the scientific efficacy and the morality of human sterilization. The biologist Fernando Ocaranza, in a talk to the Eugenics Society in 1933 on the limits of eugenics, opposed eugenic sterilization, as did several other physicians.[79] The following year, the new Nazi eugenic sterilization law was discussed at meetings during the "Second Eugenics Week" held by the society in Mexico City under the auspices of the Ateneo de Ciencias y Artes, the most distinguished of the scientific societies in Mexico. The law was roundly criticized on the grounds that knowledge of the laws of heredity was inadequate to justify such sweeping measures.[80] The feeling was, after all, that eugenic sterilization was an "anachronism" in Mexico.[81]

Matrimonial Eugenics in Comparative Perspective

Brief though the experiment in eugenic sterilization was in Mexico, it provides an interesting case study of the legislative, materialist approach to eugenics in Latin America and the conditions in which an extreme interventionist eugenics could find a place in Latin culture. The politics of eugenics in Mexico is seconded by the very different experience of Puerto Rico—seconded in the sense that the space for human sterilization for eugenic purposes depended most especially on the politics of secularism. Puerto Rico had no revolutionary ideology to sustain a rationalist, negative reproductive eugenics; it was a quasi-colonial political dependency of the United States and highly vulnerable to the imposition of conservative North American policies. By the 1930s the United States possessed the most extensive and extreme eugenic legislation in the world outside

Aninat, *Eugenesia y su legislación* [note 4], pp. 211–17, mentions that the Mexican representative to the Third Pan American Conference of National Directors of Health, held in Washington in 1936, indicated that sterilization was permitted if the Comité de Protección de la Infancia approved; he probably referred, however, to medical as opposed to eugenic sterilization. The actual application of the sterilization law needs to be researched.

79. Fernando Ocaranza, "Límites de la eugenesia," *Eugenesia* 2 (December 4, 1933): 27–29; Eliseo Ramírez, "Discurso," *Eugenesia* 2 (November 1, 1933): 19–22.

80. Alfredo Saavedra, "Relato general de los estudios presentados en la segunda semana de eugenesia," *Eugenesia* 2 (August 30, 1934): 85–89.

81. Anastasio Vergara, "El control de la natalidad desde el punto de vista de la eugenesia," *Eugenesia* 3 (October 30, 1934): 14.

of Nazi Germany, and this fact, together with political opportunity, explains the legalization of eugenic sterilization in Puerto Rico as a putative scientific-eugenic solution to the island's "overpopulation" and poverty. In 1937, under pressure from U.S. officials and against the wishes of the Catholic church as well as many people on the political left, Puerto Rico created a Eugenic Board and legalized both birth control and sterilization of those individuals deemed unfit for reproduction.[82]

Following the Nazis' institutionalization of eugenic sterilization on a massive scale in the 1930s and the revulsion against eugenics it provoked, the Latin Americans often took pride in the fact that, unlike the "Anglo-Saxons," they had not stooped to reducing human beings to mere animals. The reality was that the Latin Americans had in fact developed their own form of a negative reproductive eugenics that redefined the meaning of sexuality, gender, and race in the national state. Looking back, we are astonished less by their restraint than by far how the eugenists were willing to go in the name of racial improvement. In a time of scientific uncertainty about the laws of heredity, the eugenists talked of the desirability of making a compulsory biological inventory of the entire population in order to establish the parameters of its racial fitness; of a forcible registration of all pregnant women after the third month in order to oblige them to undergo medical monitoring and treatment; and the prohibition of marriage to "habitual drunkards." Although much of the work of the eugenists remained at the level of prescription and although their laws of negative eugenics were rarely implemented, cultural codes have effects on how individuals live their lives and interact with one another. Negative eugenics in Latin American countries was significant because it produced a set of racial and sexual ideas, prohibitions, and medical expectations that both reflected and created the gender and racial divisions within their societies.

82. Details in Annette B. Ramirez de Arellano and Conrad Seipp, *Colonialism, Catholicism, Contraception: A History of Birth Control in Puerto Rico* (Chapel Hill: University of North Carolina Press, 1983), pp. 51–55, 139.

5

National Identities and Racial Transformations

In 1921 the Mexican evolutionist Alfonso L. Herrera predicted that in the not very distant future laboratory science would allow humanity to realize on earth "the dream of Paradise," in which would reign "supreme beauty of form, intellect, and virtue." This perfect form would be, he thought, "Hellenic."[1] Some Brazilian eugenists shared that dream, imagining a time in which the Brazilian people would also be "transformed into pure Greeks."[2] These fantasies of human transmutation remind us that eugenics was above all an aesthetic-biological movement concerned with beauty and ugliness, purity and contamination, as represented in race. It was, one writer said, about "negroes, cobrizos, yellow peoples, and mestizos."[3]

Eugenics was of course a movement of "race improvement," and the relation between eugenics and racism is therefore often taken to be a defining one. But racism has many forms and is produced out of social relations in a variety of ways. Donald Mackenzie argues,

---

1. Herrera, quoted in Israel Castellanos, *Plasmogenia* (Havana: Rambla, Bouza, 1921), p. 124n.

2. Octavio Domingues, *Hereditariedade e eugenía: Suas bases, suas teorias, suas aplicações práticas* (Rio de Janeiro: Civilização Brasileira, 1936), p. 147. Domingues was criticizing some of the eugenists for their viewpoint.

3. Quote from Arturo R. Rossi, "Herencia, constitución, eugenesia y ortogénesis," *Anales de Biotipología, Eugenesia y Medicina Social* (hereafter *ABEMS*) 95 (March 1941): 16.

for instance, that in Britain class and professional interests structured the meaning of race improvement. Loren Graham shows that in the 1920s many German eugenists protested against the identification of eugenics with "race hygiene" and the theories of Nordic supremacy; Sheila Faith Weiss seconds this interpretation, characterizing German eugenics in its early years as a movement about improving national efficiency. By the late 1920s German eugenics had intertwined with anti-Semitism, and after 1933 racist eugenics became an integral part of National Socialism.[4] In the United States eugenists were preoccupied by "poor whites" at home and "inferior" immigrants from abroad; class fears and racist projections were thus both integral to the movement.[5]

These examples show that the racism of eugenics varied according to contingent and local circumstances. As I said in the Introduction, races are not preexisting natural entities but social groups produced out of unequal power relations and discriminatory practices. Science has been one of the most powerful languages for representing races because it is a language of nature and because scientists' claim to objective knowledge conceals the political processes of boundary-setting which construct races as "natural" groups.

The distinctive interest of Latin American eugenics and its racism lies in part in the particular orientation the eugenists brought to science. As we have seen, many eugenists grounded their ideas on Lamarckian theories of heredity. One of the attractions of Lamarckism as a theory was that it was believed to be inherently antiracist. For instance, a Salvadorian, Francisco Peña Trejo, complained about the racism of Galtonian eugenics as he had heard it expressed at the second International Eugenics Congress in New York; he contrasted British, Darwinian ideas of inequality with French Lamarckian egalitarianism.[6] Of course, biology is in fact never univocal, and

4. See Donald E. MacKenzie, *Statistics in Britain, 1865–1930: The Social Construction of Scientific Knowledge* (Edinburgh: Edinburgh University Press, 1981); Loren Graham, "Science and Values: The Eugenics Movement in Germany and Russia in the 1920s," *American Historical Review* 83 (1977): 1135–64; and Sheila Faith Weiss, *Race Hygiene and National Efficiency: The Eugenics of Wilhelm Schallmayer* (Berkeley: University of California Press, 1987).

5. See Nicole Hahn Rafter, ed., *White Trash: The Eugenic Family Studies, 1877–1919* (Boston: Northeastern University Press, 1988); Garland E. Allan, "The Eugenics Record Office at Cold Spring Harbor, 1910–1940," *Osiris* 2d ser. 2 (1986): 225–64.

6. Francisco Peña Trejo, *Eugenesia americana en El Salvador* (San Salvador: Imprenta Nacional, 1926), p. 8.

Lamarckism could as easily lend itself to negative and racist views as to positive and antiracist ones.[7] No science escapes the political conflicts of the society in which it is produced; the study of Latin American cases allows us to explore some of the varieties in "racial Lamarckism" and the circumstances in which they developed.

Peña Trejo's remarks also alert us to the complicated processes of self-making involved in Latin American eugenics, another reason for its interest. Latin American countries were generally stereotyped negatively by European scientists as "new" nations whose identities had not yet stabilized in coherent racial forms. The Argentine people were viewed as at best poor Europeans. Mexico, with its Indians and mestizos, was considered in no way to approximate the white norm of the racists; in Brazil, the tropical climate was considered a further factor causing the deterioration of its mixed-race population.[8]

Especially damaging to Latin American self-images was the scientific view of racial hybridization, universally condemned by biologists abroad as a cause of Latin American degeneration. Latin American intellectuals were only too prone to project onto themselves—or onto fractions of themselves, which served as their own "others"—these negative judgments of the outside world. Yet there were also limits to the degree to which Latin Americans could apply to themselves a thoroughly racialized view of their own countries' capacities for civilization and progress. They asked whether racial mixture was always a sign of inferiority or a cause of national decay; whether hybridization could not have more positive biological-social meanings; whether it should rather be encouraged as a biological process of nation formation, allowing the emergence of a national homogeneous type through a process of racial fusion.

These efforts at reevaluation of the national self were carried out in the name of race, not in rejection of race as an explanatory variable of history. Eugenics was a movement of biology, and "race" was one of the "keywords" of the twentieth century.[9] Yet the need

7. Peter J. Bowler provides an interesting example in "E. W. McBride's Lamarckian Eugenics and Its Implication for the Social Construction of Scientific Knowledge," *Annals of Science* 41 (May 1984): 245–60.

8. For an analysis of these themes in racial science, see Nancy Leys Stepan, "Biological Degeneration: Races and Proper Places," in *Degeneration: The Dark Side of Progress*, ed. J. Edward Chamberlin and Sander L. Gilman (New York: Columbia University Press, 1985), pp. 97–120.

9. I refer here to Raymond Williams's *Keywords: A Vocabulary of Culture and*

to answer negative European racial mythologies about hybridization and degeneration with mythologies of their own was at times deeply felt by intellectuals and scientists and led them at times to rethink the meanings of race without giving up their commitments to an international language of human difference and inequality.

One way to rescue themselves from the charge of inevitable racial decay was to invoke the notion of "constructive miscegenation," an idea long part of European racial science but increasingly narrowly construed as European thought became more racist.[10] In France, for example, in the mid–nineteenth century, the French anthropologist Paul Broca had concluded on the basis of animal analogies that "closely allied races" could cross with eugenesic results, while "remotely allied ones" could not.[11] By these criteria, the mixture of the different stocks that constituted France and some other European nations was found to be eugenic.[12]

To Europeans, the Indian-Negro-European crosses of Latin American nations did not meet European standards of "closeness." But closeness was based not on well-established biological tests of the degree of departure from objectively established norms but on subjective, aesthetic, political judgments that were then represented as "natural." If, then, the notion of constructive mixing was adopted by Latin American scientists, it was because the idea served the needs of people in an era of extreme negative racial stereotyping. For some Latin Americans, the notion that their own racial crossing could have positive results was precisely the wedge in international biological theory which opened up racist science to their own political projects and allowed them to reclaim themselves as eugenic nations-in-the-making. These reformulations of hybrid degeneration could serve widely diverging ideological purposes. Some scientists argued that through racial hybridization the "lower races" would be absorbed into the "higher," therefore eliminating the lower and fix-

---

Society (New York: Oxford University Press, 1985). The entry appears under the heading "racial" (though the term "race" is discussed); see pp. 248–50.

10. The term has been used by several commentators on racial ideology. It was not a nineteenth-century or eugenic expression, though the idea was.

11. Paul Broca, On the Phenomena of Hybridity in the Genus Homo, ed. C. Carter Blake (London: Anthropological Society, 1864), pp. 54–60.

12. There was a good scientific reason for considering hybridization a normal and positive aspect of biological species: the hybrid vigor often seen in mixed varietals. The failure to apply the notion of hybrid vigor to human populations is a measure of the racism that pervaded science until well after World War II.

ing the national identity in the higher race. Such a formulation left the basic racist evaluations of European science intact. Others argued that the mixture of disparate racial fractions could produce a new and superior racial type. Such a formulation challenged the notion that the mestizo was, by definition, "not eugenic." Pushed far enough, such racial inversions could turn the theory of racial hybridization on its head. The eugenics movements in Latin America showed variations on these themes of race, nation, and degeneration. They are of comparative interest because they demonstrate the tensions between the international and more local dimensions of the "science of race improvement."

Argentina and a Racialized Eugenics

Argentina, as we have seen, was the most conventionally racist in its eugenic ideology. In 1918 the country considered itself to be largely white and immigrant; its black population, once quite sizable, had by the 1880s been reduced to less than 2 percent of the national population. The indigenous "Indians" were socially marginalized. Argentinians believed their country to be not at all like Mexico, which in 1911 believed itself to be 35 percent Indian, 50 percent mestizo (Indian-white) and 15 percent creole (white), or like Brazil, which was 15 percent black and 40 percent mestizo-mulatto, the rest being "whites," relatively few of whom could claim complete "purity of blood." Indeed, Argentina seemed to many Latin Americans to be the only country that had realized its elites' old dream of racial transformation by whitening and Europeanization.

But racial ideology is not, as I have argued, a matter of "racial facts" or social reality projected into the realm of ideas. Although the racial statistics of Argentina are invariably cited as the causes of Argentinian racism, those statistics were themselves social and scientific products that were given meaning and value in specific contexts.

To explain the racism of Argentinian eugenics we have to look at the changes in the construction of the nation during the 1920s and 1930s and the way these changes informed the politics of national identity. Attitudes toward immigration had already began to alter before World War I; it was then that the professional classes began to view even European immigration as a mixed blessing. Not only were the majority of immigrants poor and uneducated Latins rather than the desired northern Anglo-Saxons; many were not even that, but Lebanese, Syrians, and Russians (usually a code word for Jews), whose capacity to assimilate into an Argentinian way of life many of the old elite profoundly doubted. A social disunity caused by class, political, and cultural divisions within an immigrant society was represented in the medical and biological discourses of the day as a fatal ethnic heterogeneity that prevented the development of the social cohesion and national spirit found in European nations.

Economic and social factors exacerbated the politics of nationality in Argentina in the late 1920s and early 1930s. The number of women in the work force grew enormously, as did prostitution, illegitimacy, and female misery. The failure of many of the working-class immigrants to take up Argentinian nationality or to marry outside their own immigrant circles added to the sense among the elite that foreign "cysts" were forming in their midst, fragmenting norms and values. Meanwhile, the new middle class also challenged the traditional political system of representation. To many conservatives, it appeared that the old culture of Argentina was giving way to a threatening mix of peoples. Such fears generated xenophobia and inflamed a desire to defend a true "argentinidad" (Argentinian identity) uncontaminated by extraneous elements.[13]

These racist ideas dominated the work of the Argentine Association of Biotypology, Eugenics, and Social Medicine in the 1930s, where the notion of a national mosaic, threatening a biological unity and the prospects of a eugenic nationality, was articulated as a pressing problem of the new eugenics.[14] The connection between Italy and Argentina in eugenic ideas is especially interesting, because it has often been said that Italian Fascism had neither the racism of the Nazis nor a racist ideology of its own. It is argued that Mussolini's Manifesto of Italian Racism of 1938 was not really Italian in origin but was imposed from the outside by Nazi Germany. Or that the

13. See Sandra McGee Deutsch, *Counter-Revolution in Argentina, 1900–1932: The Argentine Patriotic League* (Lincoln: University of Nebraska Press, 1986), pp. 39–43. For a general account of racial thought in Argentina see Aline Helg, "Race in Argentina and Cuba, 1880–1930," in *The Idea of Race in Latin America, 1870–1940*, ed. Richard Graham (Cambridge: Cambridge University Press, 1990), pp. 37–69.

14. See Gregorio Aráoz Alfaro, *Por la salud y vigor de la raza* (Buenos Aires: Coni, 1915); Alfredo Verano Fernández, *Las doctrinas eugénicas (Ensayo de sistematización)* (Buenos Aires: Liga Argentina de Profilaxis Social, 1929), and his *Para una patria grande, un pueblo sano* (Buenos Aires: Liga Argentina de Profilaxis Social, 1938).

relatively small number of Jews either deported or killed in the anti-Jewish purges is evidence of the resistance of ordinary Italians to German-style racism. Recent scholarship, however, has given us a different picture of Italian racism, emphasizing its native roots in the 1920s and its particular caste.[15] "Defense of the race," meaning the defense of the white race that supposedly made up Italy, was part of Mussolini's ideology throughout the 1920s. Italian Fascists identified their civilization with a "Mediterranean" or "Latin" people; they imagined this race as a timeless essence linking the ancient world of Rome with the present, and embracing and joining together all peoples of Latin descent wherever they were found. The Italians, who tended to present this race in "spiritual" terms, liked to distinguish their ideas of race from the more reductively biological ones of the Nazis. Whatever the language, in fact, it came to much the same thing—an emphasis on unity, purity, and type as the foundation of civilization.

These ideas found a ready audience in Argentine nationalist circles. By the 1930s it was clear to the conservative eugenists and biotypologists that Argentina's identity was going to be Latin, not Anglo-Saxon. A positive assessment of this Latin identity was under way, in opposition to the "marginal" others migrating to the cities from the Argentine countryside and from abroad. This reassessment took several forms—a revival of interest in national history, nostalgia for Hispanic cultural roots, insistence on Spanish as the language of education, and even rehabilitation of the Indian as a romantic element of Argentina's past. The eugenists' contribution to the nationalist moment was to give biological currency to the idea of Latinity and thereby new life to scientific racism.[16]

According to its president, Arturo R. Rossi, the Association of Biotypology, Eugenics, and Social Medicine was dedicated to "defending white civilization . . . with energy and tenacity" against the "profound polymorphism of our people."[17] To the eugenists, the immigration that many Argentines had welcomed as a way of swelling the population and providing the cheap labor necessary for

15. For an interesting analysis of some of the Italian Fascist writing on race in the 1920s and 1930s, see Risa Sodi, "The Italian Roots of Racialism," *UCLA Historical Journal* 8 (1987): 40–70.
16. See Nicolás Pende's "Biología de las razas y unidad espiritual mediterránea," *ABEMS* 3 (April 1, 1935): 2–4; and Helg, "Race in Argentina and Cuba" [note 13].
17. Rossi, "Herencia, constitución, eugenesia y ortogénesis" [note 3].

economic growth was producing a terrible "ethnic mosaic." The eugenists argued that their country's potential for a true Latin identity was threatened by incommensurable fractions of non-Latin peoples who had no settled race and whose crossings with the Argentinian type would dilute the national identity of the country.

Rossi maintained that the chief problem facing Argentina was that it had no certain nationality. The country was not one people but a mixture, an amalgam, or worse, a "superimposition" of various ethnic and racial elements that had failed to come together in any kind of biological unity. Members of the association believed immigration without eugenic and racial selection to be profoundly damaging to the nation-state; it was allowing in non-Latin, "Asian" or "Oriental" races, such as the Syrians and Lebanese, people weighed down by psychic and physical defects. These "sins against eugenics," it was argued, needed the remedy of tough immigration laws that took into account the eugenic fitness of individuals and their race.

These anti-immigrant and selectionist views were underscored by the eugenically oriented immigration law passed in the United States in 1924 and by the search for a Pan American code of immigration and migration control in the region in the early 1930s. The majority of the Argentinians in the association rejected eugenic sterilization but admired the United States's racial segregationist and eugenic immigration policies. The Argentine jurist Carlos Bernaldo de Quirós, for whom the racial issue became an obsession, recommended excluding altogether Jews, Poles, mulattos, and "zambos" (crosses between Indians and Negroes)—the first two types for reasons of "cultural" incompatibility, the latter two for "racial" ones. He advised against interracial marriages; in the circumstances, his condemnation of the Nazis' Nuremberg racial law against the Jews seems completely hollow.[18]

By the early 1940s, the discourse of biotypology and eugenics was shifting toward more demographic-statistical concerns (an orientation in eugenics which characterized Italian eugenics generally). The equation of state, race, and civilization was complete. When Rossi looked at Argentina, he saw a nation that was essentially white in

18. Gregorio Aráoz Alfaro, "Nuestros problemas eugénicos: Verdades dolorosas," *Hospital Argentina* 3 (November 30, 1932): 516–19; and Carlos Bernaldo de Quirós, *Problemas demográficos argentinos* (Buenos Aires: Cruz del Sur, 1942), and *Eugenesia jurídica y social (Derecho eugenésico argentino)*, 2 vols. (Buenos Aires: Editorial Ideas, 1943).

comparison with Brazil. Rossi's main concern was that the fertility coefficient of the white race in Argentina was low, a state of affairs he blamed on the liberalism, individualism, hedonism, and democratic values of so many Argentinians. The power of the state depended on the size and fertility of its race, and the Argentinian state therefore needed to control the ethnicity and race of its people.[19]

Given the racist outlook of the association and its ties to Italian Fascism, it is interesting to inquire whether the association was anti-Semitic and what the members made of the new eugenic and racial laws of Nazi Germany. The answer to these questions may help place eugenics politically, since anti-Semitism was characteristic of a particular stream of right-wing thought in Argentina in the 1930s. The Jews were stereotyped in everyday life and in the right-wing press as an alien race; they were said to bring with them dangerous and unfamiliar ideas, such as communism, and strange languages and customs. They were seen as disturbing elements, fundamentally foreign.

Somewhat suprisingly, anti-Semitism surfaced rarely or only indirectly in the association's journal, although the issue was not totally absent. The Jews were usually not named as such but were referred to indirectly as the "Russian," "eastern," or "Oriental" type whose language, customs, and habits made them an unassimilated and unassimilable element in the Argentine nation. In general, the manifest hostility to the Jews in Argentina among Catholic and conservative groups was explained away as a matter of "culture" rather than race. This self-justification was of course commonplace and could hardly be taken at face value.

On one occasion anti-Semitism erupted directly into the proceedings of the association; this eruption came at the moment when the Nazi government was putting its anti-Jewish policies in place. On October 15, 1934, the editor of the association's journal received from Justus Brinckmann, described as the head of the "German" section of the association, a copy of a lecture that had been given by the German minister of the interior, titled "The Racial Legislation of the Third Reich." Its aim was to defend the new anti-Semitic legislation of Nazi Germany against criticism, especially by German Jews who had been forced into exile. The minister claimed that the racial laws were designed to "reassert the dominance of the Aryan" rather

19. Rossi, "Herencia, constitución, eugenesia y ortogénesis" [note 3].

than to impugn the value of "other races." The editor of the journal published the article without editorial comment beyond the statement that the passionate interest racial matters were arousing at the time justified its printing.[20]

Three months later, the editor let his readers know that the article had created a very bad impression in some circles, especially in New York, as was evident from a letter received by the vice president of the association, Gonzalo Bosch, from Franz Boas, the anthropologist and outspoken critic of scientific racism, and William White, president of the International Committee for Mental Hygiene. Boas's attention had been drawn to the article by a young Argentinian anthropologist in Buenos Aires, David Efron, who was connected to Columbia University and who had asked Boas to reply to the article. The editor was thus forced to publish Boas's denial of the scientific truth of National Socialist ideas about race and therefore of the scientific legitimacy of the Nazi legislation.[21] The president of the association then announced a ban on all further discussion of the matter in the journal, since the "violent emotions" it aroused in readers prevented them from examining it objectively and scientifically, as he said Professor Boas had done. He agreed, however, to print one last word from David Efron, who protested "as a Jew and as an Argentinian" against Brinckmann's effort to insert anti-Semitism into the association. And there the matter ended.[22]

This episode was the only one of its kind I have encountered in the Argentine association's publication. The absence of more explicit demonstrations of anti-Semitism within the association, however, does not of course necessarily mean its absence in thought and action. Indeed, the extraordinary silence in the Argentine Association of Biotypology in regard to German eugenic racism—the absence of a repudiation—speaks volumes. Racism is as much a matter of daily social practices and unspoken agreements as of overtly expressed intellectual discourse or social ideology. Discretion often stops certain things from being said in public even when they are assented to in private. Although we cannot know the private thoughts of the eugenists in Argentina in the 1930s, the cordial relations between

20. "La legislación racista del Tercer Reich," *ABEMS* 2 (October 15, 1934): 12–14.

21. "La legislación racista," *ABEMS* 2 (January 15, 1935): 6–8.

22. "Arias y no arias," *ABEMS* 2 (February 1, 1935): 18.

them and Fascist Italy, the existence of a German section within the association, and the pervasiveness of racism in general in the other writings of the eugenists suggest that anti-Semitism was an unspoken aspect of their racial ideology.

The "Cosmic Race" and Mexican Eugenics

Mexican eugenists took an almost diametrically opposite line on race to that taken by the Argentinians. Yet underlying this difference were very similar preoccupations with the makeup of the imagined community of the "nation."

Of course, the traditional Indian population of Mexico was itself a political-racial construction; the rural population was divided into many groups, each with its own language and culture. Their social and cultural ties were intensely local. Even in the 1920s, many of them did not think of themselves as part of a single Indian culture or a national Mexican one, as government officials learned with surprise when they discovered, as Shirley Brice Heath says, that a great many people "had no broader concept of 'fatherland' than the village in which they had been born."[23] The idea of a Mexican people, united culturally and linguistically and bound by common goals and customs, seemed far from being a reality.

Yet the Mexican elite strongly felt the political need to answer negative European racial mythologies with mythologies of their own. Martin S. Stabb has shown that a process of modification of European science through "racial inversion" began in Mexico well before the Mexican Revolution.[24] It was particularly noticeable in the days of Porfirio Díaz, when evolutionism and scientism were popular among intellectuals. Justo Sierra and other thinkers tended to reject the excessively negative judgments about Spanish America's destiny made by such European writers as Gustave Le Bon and replace them with more positive views of the mestizo as the dynamic element in national life. In a brilliant assessment of the idea of race in Mexico, Alan Knight has linked these racial myths to the development model espoused by the elite: the land-bound Indians would be replaced by

23. Shirley Brice Heath, *Telling Tongues; Language Policy in Mexico, Colony to Nation* (New York: Teachers College Press, 1972), p. 86.
24. Martin S. Stabb, "Indigenism and Racism in Mexican Thought, 1857–1911," *Journal of Inter-American Studies* 1 (1959): 405–23.

a mobile, urban, and modern labor force made up of mestizos. Other Mexican writers in the same period, such as Andrés Molina Enriques, were less enthusiastic in their endorsement of the mestizo, yet even he agreed that the mestizo had sufficiently good qualities to allow Mexico a positive future.[25]

It is with the Mexican Revolution, however, that we witness the full development of counterracial mythologies. The first decade of the revolution, from 1910 to 1920, unleashed a social upheaval of unprecedented scale and violence; the opportunities for institutionalization of the revolution itself, and of intellectual and cultural life, were small. The fires of rebellion and protest continued to flare throughout the 1920s, and some of the largest peasant rebellions broke out then. Nevertheless, under President Alvaro Obregón, who came to office in 1920, the revolution entered what is now recognized as its "statist" period, in which a new political, cultural, and social consensus was established, often with force, sometimes through education, and through the creation of new symbolic discourses.

We associate the 1920s with the flowering of the symbolic discourse of *indigenismo*—the "sympathetic awareness of the Indian," as Stabb puts it, as a cultural sign of the Mexican nation. This official *indigenismo* had little to do with a real appreciation of the contribution of Indian cultures to the revolution or with a determination to make the Indian peoples truly the center of a social revolution. It was rather a discursive gesture of a European-oriented elite, a gesture, Knight suggests, made easier by the fact that the Mexican Indians had no unified consciousness of themselves as Indians or unified political projects of their own. *Indigenismo* was, as Knight says, a construction of the Indian by the white elite, and one that carried with it no profound commitment to social reforms.[26] It led to anthropological and sociological studies of the Indians, to the excavation of the great archeological monuments of the Indians' past, and to a romanticized celebration of their roles in Mexican culture and literature. But nowhere did it celebrate the autonomy and independent value of the variety of Indian peoples, languages, habits, cus-

25. Alan Knight, "Racism, Revolution, and *Indigenismo*: Mexico, 1910–1940," in *Idea of Race in Latin America* [note 13], pp. 71–113.
26. Stabb, " Indigenism and Racism" [note 24], p. 405; Knight, "Racism, Revolution" [note 25].

toms, or ways of life as permanent aspects of the future consolidated Mexican nation.

That role was left for the mestizo, and it was *mestizaje* (or racial amalgamation) that became the unoffical ideology of the Mexican state in the 1920s and early 1930s. One of the most famous celebrators of constructive miscegenation in Mexico was José Vasconcelos, a prolific essayist and mythmaker who, having been converted to the cause of the revolution in 1917, served under General Obregón first as rector of the reestablished National University and then as the minister of education in the 1920s, and who in these capacities identified the mestizo as the vital national element of Mexican life.[27] It was an identification found in the work of the anthropologist Manuel Gamio, as well as in that of many others whose political-ethnic ideal was to assimilate all the racial elements of the nation into a single cultural and biological norm.[28]

In two popular if controversial essays, *The Cosmic Race* (1924) and *Indianology* (1925), Vasconcelos developed the idealization of *mestizaje* more fully than anyone had done before. Vasconcelos imagined Latin America as providing the stage for the rise of a new age, dominated by a new and "cosmic" race. It would be new because it would represent a final stage of race formation, the yellow and white races having had their moment of dominance on the world stage. It would be cosmic because all races would be fused in a new racial unity. It would be Latin American because it was in Latin America that all races were already present and the process of racial fusion had already been furthest advanced. Last, the cosmic race would be tropical, because all great civilizations had been born in the tropics.[29]

Here is a fascinating instance of the use of constructive miscegenation and the inversion of the valuations built into European and North American racism to create a satisfactory myth of nationhood at a time of profound social disunity and political turbulence. The

27. See Gabriella de Beer, *Vasconcelos and His World* (New York: Las Americas, 1966) for details of his life.

28. On Gamio see the very interesting analysis by David A. Brading, "Manuel Gamio and Official Indigenismo in Mexico," *Bulletin of Latin American Research* 7(1) (1988): 75–89. Brading stresses Gamio's modern, secular commitment to a homogeneous nation based on *mestizaje*.

29. See José Vasconcelos, *La raza cósmica: Misión de la raza iberoamericana* (Paris: Agencia Mundial de Librería, 1944), esp. the prologue. There are numerous editions of this work.

despised racial mixture was now praised and the tropical climate prized as a source of excellence. Vasconcelos dismissed the racist writings of Herbert Spencer and Gustave Le Bon as the typical slanders of imperialists and presented himself as an "apostle of pariahs, advocate of clients who had no faith in their own cause."[30] "In the new phase of history that we are now in," he wrote, "we must reconstitute our ideology and organize ourselves according to a new ethnic doctrine for our entire contintent. Let us begin therefore by making our own life and our own knowledge. If we do not liberate our spirit, we will never liberate matter."[31] In *Indianology* he reported that when he proclaimed the advent of the cosmic race to a large mulatto audience in Santo Domingo, he was applauded as though he were some kind of messiah.[32]

Vasconcelos seemed to sum up the degree to which the Mexican revolutionary intelligenstia was willing to set itself in opposition to the racist-eugenic norms of other countries. The Argentinian eugenist Bernaldo de Quirós acknowledged that the Mexican ideal was indeed the opposite of the Argentinian.[33] This difference did not mean, however, that Vasconcelos repudiated eugenics per se. On the contrary, Vasconcelos, in keeping with his education as a man of science and letters, adopted the language of eugenics; but as with racial theory, he redesigned it to suit his own ends. Vasconcelos explicitly rejected what he called "scientific eugenics," or "physiological eugenics," which led to doubt about the value of racial crossings. In its place he imagined a far superior *spiritual eugenics*, a "mysterious eugenics of aesthetic taste," which would lead the beautiful and healthy individuals of each race to seek mates like themselves. The ugly, the monstrous, the abnormal—the Mendelian "recessives," as he dubbed them (showing an inadequate grasp of genetics)—would not be chosen for procreation and would eventually naturally disappear from the population. The result would be

30. Quoted in Beer, *Vasconcelos and His World* [note 27], p. 293. Vasconcelos made the perspicacious comment that the adoption by the dominant (white) race of a pseudoscientific attitude to justify its imperialistic activities had the effect of making the subjugated believe in their own inferiority. He added that this feeling had to be uprooted (p. 300).

31. Vasconcelos, *Raza cósmica* [note 29], pp. 33–44.

32. Quoted in Beer, *Vasconcelos and His World* [note 27], p. 79.

33. Quirós, *Eugenesia jurídica y social* [note 18], 1:225.

that, under socialism, a racial type infinitely superior to those that had previously existed would prevail, not just because in it were fused all the races of the human family, but because in it were conjoined only the superior individuals of all the races. The cosmic race, in short, would be a eugenic, mestizo race.[34]

Like so many of the revolutionary myths that have acquired cultural hegemony in Mexico, the idea of the cosmic race has proved highly resistant to demythologization. It has tended to be taken at face value rather than examined critically, as though a commitment to the mestizo meant an actual acceptance of all and every race in the nation, or even a devaluation of racial biology in Mexican history. The opposite is really true. It is important to recognize the degree to which Vasconcelos's idealization was fundamentally structured by the racism of the period. Putting aside Vasconcelos's turn to the right in the 1930s and his repudiation of these ideas, we see that even his earlier statements reflected the overwhelming importance attached to biological race as a factor in social life. There were limits, too, to how far Vasconcelos was willing to push the notion of "constructive miscegenation," limits that can also be seen as reflecting anxieties about Mexico's racial identity.[35]

These same kinds of anxieties were expressed within the eugenics movement of the 1930s, which both denied and asserted the significance of race to Mexico's future. As we have seen, eugenics surfaced more prominently in the 1930s than at any time before; in Mexico the decade was a time of intensified nationalism, of the formation of new structures to organize the workers, and the institutionalization of the revolutionary party, PRI (Partido Revolucionario Institucional). Within eugenics groups, the concern for racial consolidation and the fitness of the Mexican nation was a prominent theme. First, we note their reverse racism and its structuring by the dominant form of racial analysis. Just as Vasconcelos had been far from substi-

34. Vasconcelos, *Raza cósmica* [note 29], esp. pp. 28–31. Vasconcelos used the language of Mendelism, not of neo-Lamarckism, to describe his idea of eugenics.

35. Vasconcelos wrote, for instance, of the inferior races becoming less prolific as they educated themselves, and the best specimens ascending in this way up the scale of ethnic improvement. See his *Raza cósmica* [note 29], p. 31. In the 1930s Vasconcelos turned from anticlericism to the defense of Catholicism and became a Hispanophile. He took Argentina as his ideal because it was the most Spanish country of Latin America and largely European. See Beer, *Vasconcelos and His World* [note 27], pp. 252–53.

tuting a purely social explanation of Mexican life for a biological one, similarly, the members of the Mexican Eugenics Society of the 1930s tended to discuss Mexican nationality in terms of race—as a matter of Indians, Europeans, and mestizos. Their main concern was with the Indians, the indigenous masses whose poverty and marginalization the eugenists recognized.

Second, the Mexican eugenists generally accepted the dominant, revolutionary ideology concerning the biological-racial virtues of racial mixing.[36] Indians, that is, were not to be excluded, biologically or culturally, from the germ plasm of the nation; eugenics was indeed seen as providing the means by which they might be included. Dr. Eliseo Ramírez, for instance, said the separation of classes and races found in other countries went against the Mexican eugenic ideal; he remarked that though it was true that some mixes could reduce the best qualities of the forebears, it was also true that hybridization could have excellent results, as the Russian geneticist Nicolay Ivanovich Vavilov had shown.[37]

Centering Mexican nationality on the mestizo, however, meant at the same time a depreciation of the Indian as an acceptable part of the national fabric. Shirley Brice Heath has remarked that the glorification of the mestizo both "admitted and denied" Indians. It admitted them as long as they adapted to modernity and adopted the rationalism and materialism of the Mexican state; it denied them as long as they clung to their traditional customs. The eugenic goal was not to give value to the variety of biological and cultural types that made up the Mexican nation but to eliminate heterogeneity in favor of a new homogeneity, the Europeanized mestizo.

Here again the eugenists followed Vasconcelos, for he had gone so far as to predict that the systematic development of an aesthetic eugenics would make the Negro race disappear completely, by a progress of negative, voluntary, aesthetic "eugenization." No one would choose to mate with a race that was by definition inferior, or

36. One exception was the medical thesis by José Eduardo González, *Algunas consideraciones sobre eugenética* (Mexico City: Companía Editora Latino Americana, 1923), in which he argued (pp. 83–85) that it was not suitable to fuse whites with the aboriginal Indians because the number of whites would then decline. His preferred method of eugenization was therefore to encourage white immigration.

37. Eliseo Ramírez, "Discurso," *Eugenesia* 2 (November 1, 1933): 19–22.

"with types whom the instinct for beauty will signal as fundamentally recessive and unworthy of perpetuation."[38]

Eugenists in the Mexican Eugenics Society had ideas somewhat similar to Vasconcelos's about the Indian. They saw the process of racial eugenization through mixing primarily as a way of elevating the Indian and other "inferior" types to the "superior" standards of the Europeanized mestizo. With the exception of the anthropologist Manuel Gamio, almost none of the eugenists maintained that fusion with the Indians would provide benefits for the Europeans.[39] Several eugenists, furthermore, expressed reservations about whether all Indians were ready to be fused with the creoles. The biologist José Rulfo expressed his opinion that racial fusion could occur only if the economic level of the Indians was raised to that of the creoles— economic distance, as it were, foreclosing true biological mergers.[40] Equality with diversity was far from being the eugenic goal. As Rulfo put it, the aim was rather to create *one racial type*.[41] The subtext of Mexican constructive miscegenation was in fact a worry that the dream of a single cosmic race—of a biopolitical homogeneity— was very far from being achieved. Vasconcelos described Spanish America as being in a state of "racial chaos"; the cosmic race was only a "stock in formation." It seems obvious that *mestizaje* was a fantasy of national unity which did almost as much to mystify the very real cultural, social, class, and political divisions of Mexican society as the Europeans' reverse theory of hybrid degeneration did to mystify their own divisions.

The worry about ethnic unity versus disunity, a worry that brought Mexican eugenics closer to Argentinian eugenics than is at

38. Vasconcelos, *Raza cósmica* [note 29], p. 31. Elsewhere Vasconcelos indicated that all races had their own superior qualities, the Negro's being that of spirituality. The contradictory nature of Vasconcelos's tales of racial destiny and identity in the Americas points to the impossibility of using European scientific models for Latin American revolutionary purposes.

39. Manuel Gamio, in "Algunas consideraciones sobre la salubridad y la demografía en México," *Eugenesia* new ser. 3 (February 28, 1942): 3–8, argued that only by intense mixing with Indians could the Europeans in Mexico gain the advantages the Indians had acquired in their adaptation to Mexico's climate and geography through centuries of harsh natural selection. This strategy, he maintained, would be sound not only politically and economically but biologically as well.

40. José Rulfo, "Ponencia de eugenesia," *Eugenesia* new ser. 3 (May 1942): 23.

41. José Rulfo, "Discurriendo sobre el individuo en la biotipología," *Eugenesia* 3 (May 30, 1935): 41.

first apparent, was most clearly expressed in the Mexican eugenists' concern about immigration. Eugenics in the 1930s followed in the wake of the tightening of immigration laws in the United States and the introduction of racial quotas and eugenic tests of fitness. The control of the flow of individuals and races across national frontiers was very much an issue, therefore, in the relations between countries, and reactively many Latin American eugenists incorporated it as a theme of their own movements. Race improvement through the control of immigration had the added advantage that it did not involve direct intervention in reproduction, and so was a much more acceptable and seemingly practicable proposition than reproductive eugenics. Especially in the years of the Depression, almost no one, it seemed, was prepared on principle to protest the exclusion of individuals or even groups from the various Latin American countries.

Vasconcelos had acknowledged that at times Latin American countries had indeed closed their doors to certain races, as Anglo-Saxon nations had done. The main reason, he said, was economic, but he also provided a biological-racial explanation—Orientals were excluded, for example, because they tended to reproduce faster than the indigenous Indians and mestizos and because repugnance to certain fusions of races existed in the region. The idea hinted at was that new races from the outside might disturb the process of unification at home.[42] In the 1920s, the government of Mexico had also rejected a proposal to settle 50,000 U.S. blacks in the Isthmus of Tehuantepac; the secretary of state said later that black immigrants would be prejudicial to Mexico because they would complicate, rather than improve, the ethnic problem. Sinophobia had also been strong in the 1920s; though there were probably fewer than 40,000 Chinese in Mexico in 1910, says Knight, the fear of economic competition produced a campaign for their expulsion "conducted with all the panoply of xenophobic racism."[43]

Among the Mexican scientists of the 1930s, immigration selection on economic and biological grounds was a persistent theme, especially in the mid- to late 1930s, when the Depression was taking its toll and when emigration of Mexicans to the United States was re-

42. Vasconcelos, *Raza cósmica* [note 29], p. 17.
43. See Charles C. Cumberland, "The Sonora Chinese and the Mexican Revolution," *Hispanic American Historical Review* 40 (1960): 191–211; and Knight, "Racism, Revolution" [note 25], p. 96.

duced. The eugenists were clearly less fired with radical enthusiasm and had moved to a much more exclusionary position. Some wanted to make sure that only the fit entered to mix their blood with the new Mexican type that was in formation. In 1933 Adrián Correa proposed that the national government set up an institute of genetics to study the ethnology of the country and to oversee immigration from the genetic point of view. Rafael Carrillo also wrote frequently on Mexico's need for some kind of eugenic immigration law, on the grounds that immigration without ethnic selection would disturb the ethnic identity of the nation. He was very negative about the Japanese, Syrians, and Lebanese, because he believed they would fail to amalgamate and assimilate and that they would therefore cause further fragmentation of the nation.[44] Alfredo Valle saw no advantage to Mexico in allowing Russians, Poles, or Czechs to immigrate, because they did not mix well with nationals but kept to their own castes, thereby refusing to contribute to the process of *mestizaje*.[45] Others were more frankly exclusionary, especially by the late 1930s; the "cosmic" race was not to be so cosmic or universal after all.[46]

Eugenics, Race, and Nation in Brazil

The Brazilian eugenics movement of the 1920s provides a particularly interesting case study of the interaction of science with social ideology. In a society that was socially hierarchical and racially stratified, Brazil's overt racism waxed and waned according to the con-

44. Adrián Correa, in *Eugenesia* 28 (July 18, 1933): 3; and Rafael Carrillo, "Tres problemas mexicanos de eugenesia: Etnografía y etnología, herencia e immigración," *Revista Mexicana de Puericultura* 3 (November 1932): 1–15, and "La población mexicana y la eugenesia," *Revista Mexicana de Puericultura* 3 (September 1934): 783–802.
45. Alfredo Valle, "La población mexicana y la eugenesia," *Eugenesia* new ser. 1 (March 1940): 11–16. J. Espinosa Masaque, *Eugenesia y enfermedades de la infancia* (Mexico City: Atlante, 1941), p. 15, went so far as to caution against certain racial mixtures altogether on the grounds that they were negative in their influence; these mixtures included Franco-Senegalese, Anglo-Rumanian, and French-Vietnamese, among others.
46. See, e.g., the editorial on the matter in the Mexican journal *Eugenesia* new ser. 1 (November 1939): 2–3, which argued that *mestizaje* could be realized for the present only by crosses between groups of white immigrants and mestizos of high economic status.

tingencies of nationalism and immigration. As a result, eugenics was pulled in different directions at different moments.

In the 1920s a reformulated *ufanismo* (exaggerated pride in Brazil) was characteristic of the intelligenstia. There was a resurgence of nationalism with the expectation that the rapid expansion of an export economy based on coffee, immigration, and the rise of new professional groups would reform the traditional politics of the nation and launch Brazil as a world power.[47] To counter the negative assessment of Brazil's identity as a mulatto and black nation made by European and North American scientists, Brazilians claimed that their country was in the process of racial transformation and improvement. Race relations, they argued, were different in Brazil from those in the United States. How different and why were subjects of controversy, but the absence of U.S.-style legal segregation based on race (because the white elite could control social mobility by informal mechanisms, such as patron-client politics) enabled the Brazilians to claim that their national character was based on "the cordial man" (o homem cordial)—the warm, privately oriented man, at ease with himself and with others and not given to racial intolerance.[48] The middle class was expanding and drawing into itself educated racially mixed individuals, such as the writer Antônio Machado and the scientist Juliano Moreira, director of the National Mental Asylum and honorary president of the League of Mental Hygiene, where eugenics was often discussed. By the 1920s the educated class was increasingly "assimilationist" in public discourse, even if privately and in their social relations racist and discriminatory.

In this context Brazil's own version of "constructive miscegenation" began to play a more positive part in the nationalist ideology. A detailed study of the "whitening" thesis in Brazilian thought has been given by Thomas E. Skidmore, who makes plain the connection between miscegenation and nationalism.[49] Against a background of

47. For an account of the political changes in this period, see Peter Flynn, *Brazil: A Political Analysis* (Boulder, Colo.: Westview, 1978), chap. 3.

48. Bolívar Lamounier, "Raizes do Brasil," *Revista Senhor Vogue*, April 1978, pp. 141–45.

49. Thomas E. Skidmore, *Black into White: Race and Nationality in Brazilian Thought* (New York: Oxford University Press, 1972); see also his essay "Racist Ideas and Social Policy in Brazil, 1870–1940," in *Idea of Race in Latin America* [note 13], pp. 7–36.

deep anxiety that Brazil had failed to achieve a homogeneous national type and that racial degeneration menaced the nation, the notion that the country's racial mixing should be seen in positive rather than negative terms began to take hold. The few pure Negroes and indigenous Indians who remained were disappearing, social thinkers argued, because both natural and social selection worked against lower types and because their high mortality rates and low reproductive rates diminished their population. Meanwhile, white immigration was seen as a vehicle for rapidly increasing the proportion of whites, while crosses between mulattos and whites favored a steady whitening because of the whites' biological superiority and because mulattos preferred partners whiter than themselves.

As early as 1911 a scientific defense of this "whitening" thesis had been provided by the director of the National Museum, João Batista Lacerda, in a paper prepared for the First Universal Races Congress in London. In 1912, Lacerda calculated from the Brazilian census data that by the year 2012 the Negro population would be reduced to zero and the mulatto to only 3 percent of the total.[50] A later statement of the whitening thesis was given by the aristocratically minded sociologist F. J. de Oliveira Vianna. Calling Joseph Arthur de Gobineau and Georges Vacher de Lapouge men of "mighty genius" for their insistence on the significance of race to civilization, he argued in his book *Meridional Populations of Brazil* (1920) that in Brazil, through the "regressive influence of ethnic atavisms" and through the crossing of mulattos with whites, over time the mulatto strain would be filtered out and whites would develop a clear biological predominance over Negroes and mestizos.[51]

Once again, this was a formulation of the "race problem" by elites confident that their own dominance and control of a black and mulatto country was secure. Brazil was an extremely hierarchical society in the 1920s, with a very limited franchise. The large white immigration to the southern, least black parts of Brazil in the last decade of the nineteenth century and the first two decades of the twentieth played its part in suggesting to the elites that blackness would be transformed into whiteness, as did the extraordinarily high mortality rates among the poor black and mulatto populations. The intelligentsia's faith in the power of whiteness to dominate over black-

50. See Skidmore, *Black into White* [note 49], p. 67.
51. See ibid., p. 200.

ness was reinforced by the continued use of informal mechanisms of social control over black mobility, as well as more institutionalized forms of repression such as the use of the police to keep the social and racial "order."

In short, publicly expressed doubts about the racial situation in Brazil were giving way to a cautiously optimistic but nonetheless racial interpretation of the social problem, which influenced the ways in which the new science of eugenics entered into scientific discourse and social debate. The whitening myth clearly rested on an idealization of whiteness; it represented the wishful thinking of an elite in control of a multiracial society in an age dominated by racism—a yearning for a real sentiment of Brazilianness in a country divided by race and class. It was a reassurance that "aryanization" (to use a word popularized in Brazil by Vianna) could be a reality in Brazil, and that the country's racial history was no impediment to a sound future.

As the whitening thesis gained ground in the 1920s, many Brazilians turned their attention away from racial pessimism and toward education, social reform, and sanitation as answers to the "national problem." For instance, Belisário Penna, the honorary vice president of the São Paulo Eugenics Society, was a political conservative and a critic of what he saw as the corrupt politics of the republic and its misguided faith in democracy and egalitarianism. As a student at the Oswaldo Cruz Institute in 1913, he had taken part in a medical expedition in the backlands of Brazil, recording the devastations caused by hookworm, Chagas disease, malaria, and malnutrition among the racially mixed, poverty-stricken people of the northeast. The journey turned Penna into a propagandist for rural sanitation and the social regeneration of the country. His book *The Sanitation of Brazil* was a vitriolic condemnation of government inaction in the field of health and the relief of poverty, and it made him a well-known figure in medical circles. To Penna, it was not race that made the *sertanejos* (people of the backlands) and *caboclos* (people of mixed Indian-Negro blood) incapable, but epidemic and endemic disease. To sanitize was, for him, to eugenize. In 1929 he reiterated his belief that social conditions were much more important to health than race or climate.[52]

52. See Nancy Stepan, *Beginnings of Brazilian Science: Oswaldo Cruz, Medical Research and Policy, 1890–1920* (New York: Science History Publications, 1976), p. 115.

Perhaps even more emblematic of eugenics in Brazil was "Jeca Tatu" (literally "backwoods hog," a term used for an armadillo and hence slang for a typical country hick), a fictional character introduced by the writer J. B. Monteiro Lobato to signify the backward condition of the Brazilian people. Jeca Tatu was poor, ignorant, dirty, and racially mixed. By 1918, however, Monteiro Lobato had changed his mind about the meaning of Jeca Tatu; in *The Vital Problem*, which he wrote expressly to popularize sanitation as a cure-all for Brazil's problems and with the desire to turn attention away from racial explanations of social disintegration, Monteiro Lobato revised his essay on the decadence of Jeca Tatu. Whereas earlier he had analyzed Jeca Tatu's degeneration as a function of his racially hybrid status, he now presented it as a result of epidemic disease. "Jeca Tatu is made, not born," he wrote.[53] If you gave Jeca Tatu food and eliminated his parasites, added Kehl, leader of Brazilian eugenics, he would become a "Jeca Bravo" (Jeca the Splendid).[54]

The Brazilian writer Fernando de Azevedo concurred. He argued that the racial composition of the country was no barrier to the success of eugenics and claimed that Jeca Tatu was one and the same as the successful *bandeirante* (armed bands) who had cleared and settled the state of São Paulo and made it great. Their differences were not racial but social and hygienic. Eugenics, he asserted, called for the elimination of poisons, not people.[55] Eugenics in the 1920s, in short, identified itself not with racism but with sanitation.

By the late 1920s, however, a more negative and racist eugenics began to circulate, for several reasons. Public uses of racism are associated with periods of social and economic turbulence, of which the 1930s was one. Greater familiarity with German and North American eugenics was another factor. The passage of the eugenically oriented immigration-restriction law in 1924 in the United States generated considerable debate in Latin America and was a theme taken up, as we have noted, in both Mexico and Argentina. The late 1920s also saw in Brazil the decline of liberalism and optimism, a decline hastened by the depression of the 1930s. Kehl's own German origins may have had something to do with his grow-

---

53. Quoted in Skidmore, *Black into White* [note 49], p. 271.

54. Renato Kehl, *A cura da fealdade: Eugenica e medicina social* (São Paulo: Monteiro Lobato, 1923), p. 203.

55. Fernando de Azevedo, "O segredo de marathona," *Annães de eugenía* (São Paulo: Revista do Brasil, 1919), pp. 115–35.

ing racism, as the German movement moved toward "race hygiene" in the late 1920s and early 1930s. Kehl certainly read German, and in 1929, when he established the *Bulletin of Eugenics*, he began to provide short abstracts in German of articles he had published in his magazine, suggesting the existence of a German readership for racist eugenics in Brazil such as could be found in the German-speaking colonies in the south and southwest. In 1929 Kehl openly praised the eugenists in Germany for their "courage" in eugenic matters, predicting that one day the state would control all reproduction (a footnote to the 1935 edition of his *Lessons in Eugenics* noted that his prediction had been borne out). Kehl also claimed later that the Central Brazilian Commission of Eugenics he founded in 1931 was modeled on the German Society for Race Hygiene (established in September of that year).

Finally, the slowing of European immigration into Brazil in the late 1920s was a factor in raising some Brazilians' concern about Brazil's racial future. Without a continual influx of white blood, what would be the result of Brazil's much-vaunted racial miscegenation? By 1933, when Kehl published his *Eugenic Fragments: Sex and Civilization* (which he called a "semiological book of genital-social ills"), he had moved far away from the idea of constructive race mixture. Kehl saw his country as a demoralized republic in search of "sound people" ("homems validos"). He was determined to draw the line more carefully between sanitation and eugenics: Brazil had less need for exercise, education, and general hygiene than for the sterilization of degenerates and criminals, the imposition of compulsory prenuptial examinations, and the legalization of birth control.[56] In the pages of the *Bulletin of Eugenics*, the language of selection, virtually absent from the Brazilian eugenics literature of the 1920s, was now much more in evidence.[57] The journal also expressed concern about the class differentials in fertility and the social costs of mediocrity and unfitness.[58] The whole tone of eugenics, as presented by Kehl and his allies, was changing, bringing it closer to the U.S. and German movements.

56. Renato Kehl, *Aparas eugénicas: Sexo e civilização (novas diretrizes)* (Rio de Janeiro: Francisco Alves, 1933), pp. 49–50.

57. See, e.g., O. Decroly, "A selecção dos bem-dotados," *Boletim de Eugenía* 1 (October 1929): 49–50.

58. E.g., Renato Kehl, "Campanha da eugenía no Brasil: Um interessante inquérito," *Boletim de Eugenía* 3(28) (April 1931): 32; and Cunha Lopes, "Pesquisas genealógicas," *Boletim de Eugenía* 3(27) (March 1931): 53–55.

Nowhere was the shift to a more pessimistic and negative eugenics more noticeable than on the subject of race. References to "our race" ("a nossa raça") were replaced by those to "the white and black races." The number of articles on the dangers of racial mixing increased in the *Bulletin of Eugenics* and dominated the later editions of Kehl's books. The journal quoted with approval the Scandinavian race scientists Jan Alfred Mjöen and Hermann Lundborg and translated selections from their writings into Portuguese.[59] Even the term "race hygiene" began to appear. Mulattos were now described as heterogeneous, unstable elements that disturbed the national order. That Brazil was attemping to achieve whitening through racial miscegenation was, to Kehl, a cause not for celebration but for sadness. Kehl advised against racial and class crossings, while insisting upon his lack of racial and class prejudice.[60]

Yet in espousing a racist eugenics so appealing to the private (and sometimes public) worries of many members of the Brazilian elite, Kehl was also writing against social and ideological currents that were pulling Brazilian eugenics in a different direction and that prevented eugenics from becoming the race hygiene movement Kehl envisaged. Several of the new, Mendelian-oriented scientists were ready to contest not only Kehl's Lamarckism but his use of eugenics for racist purposes. By the 1930s Brazilian anthropologists and social scientists could turn increasingly to an antiracist scientific tradition for arguments and evidence. While Kehl called for a negative and racist eugenics based on the transmission of acquired characteristics, some of the Mendelians called for a more voluntaristic, less racist-oriented eugenics that would work with sanitation for the improvement of the "race."

One of Kehl's critics was Octavio Domingues, a geneticist working in the state of São Paulo at the agricultural institute of Pi-

59. Jan Alfred Mjöen, "Cruzamento da raça," *Boletim de Eugenia* 3(32) (August 1931): 49–54; and Hermann Lundborg, "Biología racial," *Boletim de Eugenia* 2(14) (February 1930): 50–51, and his "Cruzamento da raça," *Boletim de Eugenia* 3(34) (October 1931): 125–27. Mjöen, leader of the popular eugenics movement in Norway, was criticized by more moderate eugenists and scientists for his views; these criticisms were aired as early as 1915, and by the time Mjöen's views were taken up in Brazil they had lost all scientific credit in their place of origin. On these points see Nils Roll-Hansen, "Eugenics before World War II: The Case of Norway," *History and Philosophy of the Life Sciences* 2 (1980): 269–98.

60. Renato Kehl, *Lições de eugenia: Refundida e aumentada*, 2d ed. (Rio de Janeiro: Brasil, 1935), pp. 136, 240–41. See also Nancy Leys Stepan, "Eugenesia, genética y salud pública: El movimiento eugenésico brasileño y mundial," *Quipu: Revista de Historia de las Ciencias y la Tecnología* 2 (September–December 1985): 351–84.

racicaba. In 1929 he argued that the Brazilian mulatto was a product of normal and healthy Mendelian hybridization, and that Brazil was a "special and precious" example of racial mixing. If the mestizo race was at times inferior, he wrote, it was no more so than the supposedly pure races of Europe. Domingues's continued commitment to the racist evaluations of the whitening ideology was revealed by his use of Mendelian genetics to argue that, on the basis of Mendelian laws governing the inheritance of skin color and Brazil's racial ratios (he believed whites outnumbered blacks), through continued racial mixture Brazilians would, over time, naturally become lighter in complexion.[61] Although ready to defend the eugenic value of birth control and even sterilization on an individual but not a racial basis, Domingues preferred a positive eugenics based on fostering a voluntary eugenic conscience in individuals through education, so that individuals with hereditary defects would refrain from reproduction. He opposed any control of reproduction by the state.[62]

Domingues's views on race and racial mixture are particularly revealing about the ways in which the whitening ideology interacted with eugenic ideology in the late 1920s and early 1930s. Domingues interpreted racial mixture not as a cause of degeneration but as a biologically adaptive process that would allow a true civilization to develop in the tropics. We see here an echo of the Mexican use of constructive miscegenation and an interesting foreshadowing of Gilberto Freyre's thesis of "racial democracy" in Brazil, with its reliance on racial biology and its positive view of race mixture as itself a form of eugenização (eugenization).

The Mendelian anthropologist Edgar Roquette-Pinto played an even more public role in keeping eugenics from being identified with strident racism at the First Brazilian Eugenics Congress in 1929. His contacts with the antiracist anthropologist Franz Boas in New York in 1926 helped to make him a defender of the value of ordinary Brazilians of all racial types. He challenged the views of Kehl, Mjöen, and others on mulatto degeneracy as not scientifically established; he also criticized Kehl's Lessons in Eugenics (which Kehl had circulated to the conference members) as not representing, in its

61. Octavio Domingues, A hereditariedade em face de educação (São Paulo: Melhoramentos, 1929), pp. 89–91, 132, 136.
62. On sterilization, see Domingues, Hereditariedade e eugenia [note 2], pp. 25–30.

more extreme opinions, the outlook of the congress.[63] Inverting
Charles Davenport's use of Mendelian genetics to warn against racial crossing in the United States, Roquette-Pinto argued that Mendelian crosses between whites and blacks were normal and healthy.[64]
He was prepared to go even further; breaking with the racist ideology of whitening, he maintained that the goal of eugenics was not
to whiten but to educate all people, black and white, to the importance of heredity, so that the eugenically minded individual, aided
by state-run programs of sanitation, would participate voluntarily in
the "purification" of the human race. Eugenics itself was based on
heredity, an area "where the state does not penetrate," he added.[65]

At the meetings of the congress, the presentation by the congressman A. J. de Azevedo Amaral on the "eugenic problem of immigration" sparked an intense debate about race and racism. Discussion
spilled over into the second and third days of the meetings, and so
heated were feelings that Azevedo Amaral's recommendations had
to be reformulated and voted on as two separate proposals: one to
restrict the entry of non-Europeans in general and another specifically to restrict the entry of blacks. Azevedo Amaral was joined in
his position by the mental hygienist Oscar Fontanelle, the clinician
Xavier de Oliveira, and the president of the National Academy of
Medicine, Miguel Couto, all of whom maintained that further racial
mixture with blacks would lead to racial degeneration. They were
opposed by Edgar Roquette-Pinto, the anthropologist Froés de
Andrade, by Belisário Penna and Fernando Magalhães, and by the
physiologist Miguel de Osorio; these men either defended racial
crossing in general or opposed immigration restriction based on ethnic or racial criteria. As president of the congress, Roquette-Pinto
played an important role in forcing the issue, which he said was a
matter not of race at all but of hygiene. Penna seconded him. Fernando Magalhães reminded the conference members that Brazil's
past was based on hybridization, adding, "We are all mestizos and

63. In his essays on Brazilian anthropology published in 1933, Roquette-Pinto
evoked the U.S. geneticist Herbert Jennings's *Prometheus Unbound* (1925) to warn
against hasty eugenists who lacked scientific data for their views: Edgar Roquette-
Pinto, *Ensaios de antropología brasileira* (1933; Rio de Janeiro: Editora Nacional, 1978),
p. 32.

64. Edgar Roquette-Pinto, *Seixos rolados (estudos brasileiros)* (Rio de Janeiro: n.p.,
1927), pp. 61–62, 174, 202.

65. Ibid., p. 205.

would therefore exclude ourselves." "We do not believe," said Froés de Fonseca, "that eugenizing the Brazilian people is a racial issue."[66]

Roquette-Pinto especially defended the eugenic worth of the Japanese as possible candidates for immigration against the attack of such scientists as Couto, who had long called for the restriction of Asian immigrants on eugenic-racial grounds.[67] Roquette-Pinto and others were willing to concede the need for some kind of individual selection of immigrants, as had been proposed in 1925 by Juliano Moreira, Pacheca e Silva, and others in the League of Mental Hygiene. What they opposed was *racial* immigration selection, which they saw as based on nothing but out-of-date, unscientific prejudice. In 1929, public racial etiquette triumphed over private racial beliefs. In a eugenics congress full of controversial subjects, Azevedo Amaral's proposals were among the few not endorsed in their original form. His demand for a national policy of immigration exclusion based on race was rejected by the participants by 25 votes to 17.[68]

Race, Nation, and Eugenics under Vargas

The following year, the First Republic of Brazil broke down in the "revolution" of 1930. The revolution was a product of new social forces, some radical in orientation, some extremely conservative, and all critical of the control of politics by the traditional and landed oligarchy. It brought to prominence Getulio Vargas, a politician from Rio Grande do Sul, who took over the presidency and prepared the way for a new constitution. These events at first seemed to promise new political and social opportunities and a space for institutional experimentation. The period saw the creation of new federal departments, notably the first Ministry of Labor. At a time when Brazil was suffering from the effects of the depression and the rapid fall in coffee prices, the collapse of established ways of doing things and the search for new ones seemed to offer the eugenists the prospect of consolidating their programs at the national level.

66. See Primeiro Congresso Brasileiro de Eugenía, *Actos e trabalhos* (Rio de Janeiro, 1929), pp. 16–42, 79, for these quotations.
67. E.g., Couto's remarks as reported in the *Boletim da Academia Nacional de Medicina* 96 (April 24, 1924): 33.
68. Ibid., pp. 20–21.

A new Central Brazilian Commission of Eugenics was established in 1931, with members drawn from the fields of public health, mental hygiene, the biological sciences, and medicine. The commission gained political visibility when one of its members, Belisário Penna, was appointed director of the Department of Health within the new Ministry of Education and Public Health. Penna's appointment gave hope to the eugenists that national antialcohol legislation would finally be introduced. In addition, Roquette-Pinto and Kehl were invited to serve on a special committee organized within the Ministry of Labor to advise on the problems of immigration.

By 1937, however, the period of tentative liberalization and limited parliamentary democracy was over. Seven years after the revolution of 1930, and only three years after the 1934 constitution was created by elected representatives, Vargas consolidated his power as the president of a new, corporatist state that lasted until 1945, when it was ended by a military coup. The Vargas period has continued to evade easy ideological and political definition.[69] Originally interpreted as a Brazilian version of European fascism, the authoritarian and corporatist Estado Novo combined a baffling mixture of regressive and progressive elements. On the one hand, after a period of political experimentation that saw the founding of the first mass parties on the democratic left (the Aliança Nacional Libertadora) and the right (the Integralista party), political repression increased, especially after 1935 and the stiffening of Vargas's control over the political system and the state. Political "dissidents" on the left and the right were policed, and eventually all political parties were suppressed and many of their leaders imprisoned.

The Vargas regime extended the power of the state to manage and control "social problem" groups such as the mentally ill, prostitutes, and juvenile delinquents. It was in this period that a state system of identity cards was discussed by the medical legal expert Leonidio Ribeiro, who opened an Institute of Identification in the federal capital in 1933 and worked closely with the right-wing police chief of the city, Felinto Muller, to bring "up-to-date," "scientific" techniques of identification and treatment of the "pathologically crimi-

69. Samuel Putnam, "Vargas Dictatorship in Brazil," *Science and Society* 5(2) (1941): 97–116, and "Brazilian Culture under Vargas," *Science and Society* 6 (1942): 34–57; Robert E. Levine, *The Vargas Regime: The Critical Years, 1934–1938* (New York: Columbia University Press, 1970); Marilena Chaui and Maria Sylvia Carvalho Franco, *Ideologia e mobilização popular* (Rio de Janeiro: Paz e Terra, 1978).

nal" to Brazil.[70] At the same time, Brazil under Vargas began to incorporate new social groups into the state, notably the urban, industrial working class, who were rewarded with new social-welfare and labor legislation in return for corporatist controls and social acquiesence.[71]

The most interesting example of the way eugenics intertwined with the new state in the 1930s concerned the formulations of race and nationality. According to Karl Lowenstein, the Vargas regime was marked by a desire to create a "homogeneous consciousness of nationhood as the basis of social and political life." New state apparatuses were developed to help create such consciousness, to mobilize patriotism, to generate a sense of national unity and to level "ethnic disparities."[72] Given this ideological orientation, deliberate public use of the language of racism, evocation of racial antagonism or difference, and public acknowledgment of the realities of racial discrimination against the black segments of the population were to be avoided (especially after Brazil entered the war against Germany in 1943). By the late 1930s, the notion that racial and cultural fusion was the solution to Brazil's racial and social makeup had become the unofficial ideology of the national state—maintained in the face of actual deep racial-class cleavages and social conflicts. National identity and homogeneity were to be encouraged by an exclusive nationalism that resulted in a series of laws restricting the number of foreigners who could hold jobs in Brazilian business firms and that made Portuguese the sole language of instruction in schools. Eventually Vargas also suppressed the use of foreign-language newspapers, foreign flags, and, insofar as he was able, the foreign identification of the German colonies in the country. In these circumstances, the racist eugenists' rejection of racial amalgamation as the answer to Brazil's identity found relatively few adherents. Fusion through racial and cultural means, enabling blackness to disappear and the nation-state to form a new homogeneity, was itself taken to be "eugenic."

On the other hand, politicians promoted immigration restriction in the 1930s not only because of the felt need to protect the national

70. Leonidio Ribeiro, "Os problemas medico-legais em face de reforma da policía," *Archivos do Instituto Médico-Legal e Cabinete de Identificação* 1 (August 1931): 11–26.

71. Flynn, *Brazil* [note 47], pp. 100–103.

72. Karl Lowenstein, *Brazil under Vargas* (New York: Macmillan, 1942), p. 193.

population from competitition for jobs during the Depression but because of growing public endorsement of a eugenically aided process of racial fusion and whitening in Brazil. The decline in European immigration in the late 1920s and the rise in Japanese immigration were critical to the eugenists' claims that Brazilianization and the forging of national unity now needed to be protected from outside threats, especially from ethnic or national groups whose physical or cultural characteristics they believed might disturb the process of racial homogenization at home. The general lament that Brazilians were still a heterogeneous people, without a clear ethnic center or sense of nationality, was, as we have seen, similar to that heard in both Argentina and Mexico, despite their different racial situations and racial ideologies. It led to an intensification of concern that groups—whether Jews, Germans, Lebanese, or Japanese—would enter the country and fail to acquire Brazilian customs, language, and habits. It was a point made by Penna at the First Brazilian Eugenics Congress of 1929, where he worried out loud about colonists who settled in large numbers and refused to adapt themselves, linguistically or culturally, to Brazilian ways.[73]

Belisário Penna had agreed in 1929 with Roquette-Pinto and other scientists involved in the debate on racial restriction that the problem was not really racial but political. But the worry about national unity—about *how* Brazil was to create a single identity and ethnicity—served to unite eugenists and politicians who otherwise had rather different outlooks on the racial issue. The breakdown of the old republic and the subsequent call for a new constitution provided the opportunity for eugenists to bring eugenic ideas about nationality and Brazilian identity into the debate about immigration. In the Constituent Assembly of 1933–1934, Couto and Oliveira rehearsed the eugenic arguments they had made in 1929 for a racial selection of immigrants. Couto's remarks were directed especially against the Japanese, 50,000 of whom had settled in Brazil that year, the largest single ethnic group to enter. Couto, who was virulently anti-Japanese, accused the Japanese of creating a "racial mosaic" in the coun-

---

73. Primeiro Congresso Brasileiro de Eugenía, *Actos e trabalhos* [note 66], p. 18. We see the expression of the same worry in Fernando de Azevedo, *Brazilian Culture: An Introduction to the Study of Culture in Brazil* (1943; New York: Macmillan, 1950), p. 37, where Japanese and German colonies are referred to as "cysts in the national organization."

try.[74] Antonio Carlos Pacheco e Silva argued that restriction was both a eugenic and a public-health measure, presenting data that purported to show that Japanese and Italian immigrants brought new diseases into the country.[75] To other members of the assembly, immigration restriction was justified by unemployment at home. From welcoming white immigration as a source of eugenization, Brazil now was about to close its doors to immigrants in the name of protecting the process of eugenization. The result of the various arguments was a eugenic and racial immigration law that established racial quotas as well as economic and other tests of fitness for entry into Brazil. These quotas were set at 2 percent of each "nationality" in the population. The policy of exclusion affected mainly the Japanese and the Jews, whom eugenists and others stereotyped as "nonassimilable" elements in the body politic; these negative images and the new selective immigration law had the effect of closing the doors to Jews fleeing Nazi persecution.[76] The immigration restriction clauses of the Constitution of 1934 were retained in the 1937 Constitution of the Estado Novo, thus ratifying the commitment to whitening, eugenization, and homogenization as the official policy of the national state.[77]

While a racist and exclusionary stand toward immigration inflows from the outside world was thus formalized by the new Brazilian constitution, within Brazil the "problem" of racial miscegenation was recast as a solution, namely "mestiçagem." As Renato Ortiz points out in his study of Brazilian culture and national identity, in place of the negative view of the lazy, indolent, and degenerate racial hybrid which had underlain nearly all discussions of Brazil's identity in the past, the positive image of the mixed-race *Brazilian*

74. Brasil, *Annães da Assembleia Constituente* (Rio de Janeiro, 1935), 4:490–93, 546–48; and Moacyr Navarro, *Miguel Couto vivo* (Rio de Janeiro: A. Noite, 1950), pp. 137–38.

75. See Teodolina Castiglione, *A eugenia no direito da familia* (São Paulo: Saraiva, 1942), p. 14.

76. See Robert M. Levine, "Brazil's Jews During the Vargas Era and After," *Luso-Brazilian Review* 5(1) (Summer 1968): 45–58. See also the detailed study of anti-Semitism in the Vargas period, and of its connection to the debates on Brazilian nationality and homogeneity, by Maria Luiza Tucci Carneiro, *O anti-Semitismo na era Vargas (1930–1945)* (São Paulo: Editora Brasiliense, 1988).

77. See Michael Mitchell, "Race, Legitimacy, and the State in Brazil," paper presented to the Latin American Studies Association, Mexico City, September 29–October 1, 1983.

was tied to a new ideology of work and modernization.[78] A myth of national identity in keeping with needs of the modern state was thereby articulated. Intellectually, the representative figure of the 1930s was the Brazilian sociologist Gilberto Freyre, not Kehl. Freyre's writings provided the key ideas that dominated domestic interpretations of Brazilian history and nationality for the next thirty years. Freyre had been trained at Columbia University, where he had come under the influence of Franz Boas and from him learned an antiracist and "cultural" orientation. Freyre also referred to Brazilian sources for his views, such as Roquette-Pinto's statement in 1929 that the Brazilian type was not racially inferior but sickly.[79] Freyre's intention was to oppose the exaggerated biological racism of such writers as Oliveira Vianna and to introduce more sociological analyses of the Brazilian "problem." In a series of classic works of Brazilian history and sociology, beginning with *The Masters and the Slaves* in 1933, Freyre emphasized Brazil's cultural diversity, defended Brazil's racial "harmony," contrasted it with the racial conflict and segregation of the United States, and argued that Brazil was unique in creating out of racial mixture a "luso-tropical" civilization in the New World.

Although in Freyre's day his writings represented a subversion of scientific racism and a critique of the racial pessimism characteristic of many intellectuals in the 1930s, they did not constitute a fundamental break with the past.[80] Freyre maintained, in effect, that far from being eugenically unfit, as Oliveira Vianna and others claimed, the Africans brought to Brazil were "eugenically" superior and had merged freely in a "racial democracy" with the Indians and with a Portuguese people culturally suited to the tropics to produce a racially mixed people of increasing ethnic and eugenic soundness.

Freyre's failure to uncover the deep racial prejudices and social practices that marginalized blacks and dark mulattos in Brazil's social system (a failure for which he was roundly criticized by a new

78. Renato Ortiz, *Cultura brasileira e identidade nacional* (São Paulo: Editora Brasiliense, 1985), pp. 36–44.
79. See Stanley J. Stein, "Freyre's Brazil Revisited: A Review of *New World in the Tropics: The Culture of Modern Brazil*," *Hispanic American Historical Review* 41 (1961): 111–13; Gilberto Freyre, *The Masters and the Slaves: A Study in the Development of Brazilian Civilization* (1933; New York: Knopf, 1963), p. xxvii.
80. See Maria Alicia de Aguir Medeiros, "Casa grande e senzala: Uma interpretação," *Dados* 23 (1980): 215–36.

generation of Brazilian social scientists in the 1960s) is not the issue here.[81] The point is that the racial and social fiction of the late 1920s and 1930s—that Brazil was a racial democracy where the various "races" intermingled freely—provided a context in which eugenics survived. The imagined community of Brazil denied the reality of racism at home and extolled the possibilities of racial harmony and unity. The variant of eugenics identified with public hygiene and compatible with racial mixing and the myth of racial democracy gained support; extreme reproductive eugenics, or Nazi-style race hygiene, did not.

Eugenics thus found itself strangely placed in Brazil in the late 1930s, its scientific and social complexion rendering any simple conclusions about the relation between science and social life impossible. Eugenics was part of national legislation, even if prenuptial tests and medical-racial tests for immigration were sporadically and inconsistently applied. Under Vargas the new labor legislation giving certain "protections" to women at work was also seen as a "eugenic" contribution to national fitness. Such words as "eugenics," "euphrenics," and "dysgenics" dotted the institutional landscape, especially in fields connected to child and maternal welfare. In the new Ministry of Labor created by Vargas in 1934 the eugenists also found a place for their ideas about fitness and national improvement; one can trace in this and other institutions a slow shift from eugenics back to puericulture and concern for infant health in the 1940s. Eugenics also continued to be evoked in the organizations concerned with juvenile delinquency, social pathology, and criminality. In the scientific field, Lamarckian-style genetics predominated in medical circles until the 1940s.[82] When the geneticist Theodosius Dobzhansky visited Brazil in the 1940s, he was surprised by the number of Brazilians who still believed in the inheritance of acquired characteristics.[83] Not until the late 1940s did Mendelism finally replace neo-Lamarckian ideas.

As Kehl and some of his associates turned in admiration to Nazi racial eugenics (without giving up their neo-Lamarckism), other

81. See especially Emilia Viotta da Costa, *Da monarchia à república: Momentos decisivos* (São Paulo: Grijalbo, 1970).

82. See, e.g., Nelson Bandeiro de Mello, "Alcoholismo e hereditariedade," *Archivos Brasileiros de Hygiene Mental* 12(3/4) (1939–1949): 84–91.

83. Theodosius Dobzhansky, *The Roving Naturalist: Travel Letters of Theodosius Dobzhansky*, ed. Bentley Glass (Philadelphia: American Philosophical Society, 1980), pp. 113, 194, 226.

Brazilian intellectuals began to discover "the Negro," and to move away from biological racism toward more culturally oriented and sociological explanations of society in which eugenics still found a place.[84] The "Manifesto of Brazilian Intellectuals against Racism," signed by (among others) Roquette-Pinto, Freyre, and the anthropologist Artur Ramos, represented the most public expression of Brazilian scientists' antiracism in the 1930s.[85]

Conclusion

In the comparative study of the history of racial eugenics, Latin America adds interesting case histories that run the gamut from overt racism to more subtle inversions of the racial ideas of Europe and the United States. As we sort out the factors that led eugenics in a more or less racist direction, certain cultural variables seem to have been relatively unimportant. The Catholic church, for instance, provided almost no restraints on racism comparable to its opposition to eugenic control of reproduction. Church criticisms of acts of discrimination and violence against the Jews in fascist countries were often feeble; when the church did protest against the Nazi laws prohibiting marriages between Jews and "Aryans," and later the equivalent laws in Vichy France, it did so insofar as they touched on the sacrament of marriage rather than in criticism of racism per se. Race was not a matter of church dogma, as marriage and reproduction were; religious faith or cultural Catholicism did not therefore restrain eugenic policies toward race.

Genetic theory also proved to be multivalent and flexibly interpreted in relation to race, with neo-Lamarckians and Mendelians lining up on the racist and antiracist sides. Obviously much more crucial in the racism of eugenics were larger, underlying social and structural factors. These determined the manner in which scientists constructed the racial identities of the nations and the attitudes they took toward the possibilities for racial degeneration or regeneration.

The espousal of "constructive miscegenation" by some eugenists was a distinctive contribution, allowing them to be part of a modern scientific movement of racial health without consigning all of Latin America to the racial dustbin of history. By the late 1930s, more-

84. Robert E. Levine, "The First Afro-Brazilian Congress: Opportunities for the Study of Race in the Brazilian Northeast," *Race* 15 (1973–1974): 185–93.
85. Artur Ramos, *Guerra e relação de raça* (Departmento União Nacional dos Estudos, 1935), pp. 177–80.

over, Latin American ideas on race crossing were becoming part of the mainstream of genetics. The historian of biology William Provine has shown that geneticists in general began to change their minds about race crossing and accept that it was a genetically normal and positive aspect of human populations. The shift in scientific opinion about race mixture, from negative to positive, owed little to developments in scientific knowledge between 1910 and 1940, says Provine, and everything to changes in political outlook.[86] Jewish scientists displaced by Hitler were especially prominent in attacking scientific racism.

When the criticisms of racism in science by the better-known geneticists, such as Hermann Muller, Herbert Jennings, Julian Huxley and J. B. S. Haldane, became known in Latin America, scientists often quoted them appreciatively and claimed that, unlike their European and U.S. counterparts, they had never endorsed an extreme racism. In some of the eugenics movements of Latin America, the countermyth of racial amalgamation had served to prevent eugenics from becoming a program of racial segregation or extermination. But though the racial valuations were changed, the structure of the eugenics argument—with its emphasis on biological differences as key factors in the making of a nation—had not. "Constructive miscegenation," it could be said, was thus as much a product of racism as its reverse. The concept had established biological race as the crux of nationhood, and left, in some instances, lasting institutional legacies in the form of immigration-restriction laws influenced by eugenics. The eugenists' emphasis on national homogenization through biological amalgamation was as much a mystification of the social and political realities of their very poor societies as was the reverse theory that warned against racial heterogeneity and hybrid degeneration. As a mode of cultural and national interpretation, biology had been put to very limited and inadequate ends, in Latin America as in any other areas of the world.

86. William B. Provine, "Geneticists and the Biology of Race Crossing," *Science* 182 (1973): 790–96.

6

U.S., Pan American, and Latin Visions of Eugenics

The scientific and medical aspects of formal and informal empire are often neglected by historians. Eugenics, for instance, was more than a set of national programs embedded in national debates; it was also part of international relations. This latter aspect of eugenics is analyzed here for the light it sheds on biopolitics in the interwar years.

A quasi-international structure for eugenics had developed early. The First International Congress of Eugenics, held in London in 1912, had been followed by a second and a third in New York in 1921 and 1932. An International Federation of Eugenic Societies had also been set up in 1921 by the head of the English Eugenics Education Society, Leonard Darwin, to coordinate the activities of eugenics organizations around the world.

Latin American contacts with these congresses and the federation were scanty, however. Far more significant to Latin American eugenics was the Pan American Union. The Pan American sanitary conferences had set a precedent for using the Pan American umbrella to foster cooperation in controlling infectious diseases that might spread from country to country. Nevertheless, Pan Americanism was primarily a U.S. idea; the headquarters of the union was in Washington, and many Latin Americans saw Pan Americanism as a vehicle for the United States to push its own point of view. In an era of growing U.S. involvement in the Caribbean and Central America, a Pan American eugenics, which touched on so many issues of national pride and power, such as the control of the flow of populations across national boundaries, was an idea perhaps predictably fraught with tensions.

The relations between Latin America and the United States were made even more problematic by the extreme nature of U.S. eugenics. From its earliest days, eugenists in the United States had taken a strongly reductionist, Mendelian line on racial improvement. The leader of U.S. eugenics, Charles Benedict Davenport, had proselytized the new eugenics under the banner of Mendelism after he visited Galton and other eugenists in England in the opening years of the twentieth century.[1] At Cold Spring Harbor on Long Island, the new experimental station Davenport founded with the express purpose of studying heredity and evolution, he pursued the theme of human heredity with relish and energy, fitting every kind of pathological condition and behavior into a highly reductive Mendelian framework.[2] The Carnegie Institution in Washington provided generous monetary support for his research; Mrs. E. H. Harriman also gave money to the Eugenics Record Office, which was begun in 1910 and directed by Davenport's deputy, Harry Laughlin. U.S. eugenics was in fact by far the best funded of all the eugenics movements.[3]

Especially difficult for the Latin Americans was Davenport's racism. According to Davenport, each race had its own fixed, biological identity. He further maintained that since, on Mendelian principles of genetics, the unit characters that determined traits in humans did not blend during reproduction but retained their independent form and persisted, in racial mixing the bad traits of an inferior type or individual would not be obliterated but rather would be preserved. In 1926 Davenport supervised a study of race crossing in Jamaica, which proved to him that racial hybrids were physiologically and psychologically inharmonious. It followed that for Davenport countries made up of racial hybrids were anathema.[4]

1. See Daniel Kevles, *In the Name of Eugenics: Genetics and the Uses of Human Heredity* (New York: Knopf, 1985), pp. 44–56.

2. See Charles E. Rosenberg, "Charles Benedict Davenport and the Irony of American Eugenics," *Bulletin of the History of Medicine* 15 (May/June 1983): 18–23.

3. In addition to Kevles, *In the Name of Eugenics* [note 1], see Barry Mehler, "The New Eugenics: Academic Racism in the U.S. Today," *Science for the People* 15 (May/June 1983): 18–23.

4. Rosenberg, "Charles Benedict Davenport" [note 2].

This was the message Davenport brought to the Pan American meetings on eugenics; in the address he prepared in 1933 for the second of them, he said: "When very dissimilar races inhabit the same country there are apt to be conflicts of interests, conflicts of mores; mutual antipathy arises, and suspicions are nurtured. There is a lack of understanding and interest or unity of principles, there arise chasms and castes."[5]

To Davenport and many of his fellow eugenists, such racial concerns led logically to the desirability of selective and restrictive immigration—to the need to keep out of the United States those dysgenic individuals and types who might overwhelm the supposedly superior American stock at home. Laughlin testified before the House Committee on Immigration and Naturalization in 1923 and 1924 on the eugenic angle and played a part in the passage of the Immigration Restriction Act (Johnson Act) of 1924.[6]

As the U.S. eugenists came increasingly to dominate international eugenics—they hosted the Second International Eugenics Congress in New York in 1921 and supplied by far the largest number of delegates and papers—there was a noticeable increase in racism in the tone and content of the papers.[7] This tendency continued into the third international conference in 1932.[8]

Their extreme reductive, racial-reproductive position made U.S. eugenists difficult partners for Latin American eugenists interested in an "American" effort that would truly include everyone in the New World. We know that the Latin American eugenists themselves were often racist in outlook; but the laws banning interracial marriages in the United States and the early adoption of racial quotas in immigration made U.S. eugenics seem much more intransigently racist than the eugenics of the Latins. Seen from a Latin American standpoint there existed another stream of eugenic interpretation and activity which was altogether milder and more practicable than the eugenics the "Anglo-Saxons" stood for. The growing economic in-

5. Quote from the typescript of Davenport's speech, June 7, 1933, Pan American Conference on Eugenics and Homiculture, in B:27, Ramos D., file 3, Davenport Papers, American Philosophical Society Library, Philadelphia. (Hereafter Davenport Papers, Ramos files).

6. See Kevles, *In the Name of Eugenics* [note 1], pp. 94–97, 102–4.

7. See *Scientific Papers in the Second International Congress of Eugenics*, vol. 2: *Eugenics in Race and State* (Baltimore: Williams & Wilkins, 1923).

8. Kevles, *In the Name of Eugenics* [note 1], chap. 11.

terest and political power of the United States in the region raised a question of which vision of eugenics—that of the United States or that of the Latins—would prevail.

The Pan American Initiative

A turning point in the relations between U.S. and Latin American eugenics came in 1921, when the Second International Congress of Eugenics was held in New York under Davenport's presidency. Eugenists in the United States had many reasons to try to stimulate the development of eugenics in Latin America and incorporate it into the United States's sphere of eugenic influence. Not the least of these reasons was Latin American racial hybridization and immigration, which to Davenport and others seemed to threaten the New World's "purity of race." As a result, several Latin American governments were invited to send delegates to the congress.[9]

Of the countries that responded, Cuba was perhaps the most important to the United States, because it was geographically close and the political connections between the two countries were strong. The United States had occupied Cuba between 1898 and 1902 and again between 1906 and 1908, and it played an important and often overbearing role in the island's economy and in the regulation of its public health. The island had a long history of racism, and the elites consistently rejected the idea of a multiracial society. Racial traditions and self-perceptions, as well as U.S. influence, played their parts in turning Cuban initiatives in eugenics in a northern direction. From the U.S. eugenists' point of view, the fact that each year hundreds of Cubans came to Florida and cities farther north was a good reason to involve the Cubans in their own "eugenization."

An opportunity to do so arose when Dr. Domingo y Ramos came to the meetings in New York from Havana. His contacts with Davenport had an immediate impact, leading him to new themes

9. See Francisco Peña Trejo, *Eugenesia en El Salvador* (San Salvador: Imprenta Nacional, 1926), p. 34, where he mentions that in addition to himself there was a Chilean delegate and a Cuban. According to Alfredo Fernández Verano, *Las doctrinas eugénicas (ensayo de sistematización)* (Buenos Aires: Liga Argentina de Profilaxis Social, 1929), p. 40, in 1915 the Eugenics Record Office asked for a commission from Argentina to represent the country at the Second International Congress, then planned to be held in 1918. World War I canceled these plans and the congress was not held until 1921.

and possibilities.[10] His thoughts focused especially on the dangers of racial crossing and immigration, themes previously absent from his writings on eugenics. The New York congress also gave Ramos the idea of creating, with Davenport's help, a new Pan American organization devoted to eugenics in which Ramos would play a prominent role. The following year the Pan American Eugenic Committee was established at the Latin American Medical Congress held in Havana, with the goal of creating a permanent Pan American Association of Eugenics and Homiculture (the title reflecting Ramos's influence and his new understanding of eugenics). At the Pan American meetings in Santiago, Chile, in 1923, the problems of heredity and eugenics were given considerable attention, and the delegates gave official approval to a new Pan American Eugenics Office, to be headed by Ramos and based in Havana.

Ramos had begun corresponding with Davenport in English as early as 1922.[11] In June of that year Ramos proposed that in reporting on the Second International Congress of Eugenics to the Cubans, he would recommend that in the future "all [eugenic] works made in Cuba shall be under your inspiration." He suggested that before any institutions were formed (Cuba had not yet created its own eugenics society), some Cubans should be sent to Cold Spring Harbor for instruction in Davenport's methods, "so that the Eugenic Station in Cuba will be in constant relation with the one in Cold Spring Harbor." He went on in his slightly awkward English: "The station in Cuba, by reasons you pointed out to me in New York—the smallness of the country and the presence of several races and also the reasons I have observed—can be of great use to the genetic researches and can also constitute the outpost for good propaganda, under your inspiration in the Latin American countries."[12]

Ramos urged Davenport to attend the First Pan American Conference of Eugenics, where Ramos planned to draw up a constitution for the organization under Davenport's presidency. "I believe

10. The paper he delivered at the congress was a brief statement of his idea of "homiculture." See D. F. Ramos "Homiculture in Its Relation to Eugenics in Cuba," in *Eugenics in Race and State* [note 7], pp. 432–34. Later he called himself Domingo y Ramos.

11. Davenport Papers, Ramos files [note 5]. There are some forty letters and typescripts relating to eugenics and Ramos's involvement with it.

12. Ramos to Davenport, June 27, 1922, Davenport Papers, Ramos files, file 1 [note 5].

you have to do, for the improvement of man's heredity in the whole America [sic], what General Gorgas did for the improvement of man's environment in the American tropics, and we shall all help you by following your ideas," he wrote to Davenport in New York.[13]

In these exchanges it was apparent that Davenport mattered more to Ramos than vice versa—that Davenport gave the Cubans the glamour and prestige they wanted. Davenport refused the presidency, advising Ramos to find someone "whose interest in eugenics may be enhanced by the office."[14] Davenport took the Pan American idea of eugenics seriously enough, nonetheless, to plan to be present at the first conference. Ramos continued to solicit Davenport's advice, particularly on immigration and race, and Davenport continued to offer it. Ramos also managed to persuade the Pan American Union that the seriousness of eugenics, and Davenport's views on immigration, justified making the Pan American Conference of Eugenics and Homiculture independent of the existing Pan American sanitary conferences.[15]

It was not until after several years of often frustrating effort (in December 1926 Ramos had to call off a meeting because of a hurricane) that Ramos's plans came to fruition and what he hoped would be the first of a series of Pan American conferences of eugenics and homiculture was held in Havana in December 1927.[16] The conference was relatively small, only twenty-eight delegates from sixteen countries attending.[17] In addition, many of those who attended were not eugenicists but diplomats from the various Latin American countries who were based in Havana and could represent their countries. From the United States, however, came Davenport himself (Richard Wilson, of the U.S. Immigration Department, failed to appear at the last minute because of illness in his family). Dr. Eusebio Hernández, hailed at the conference as the founding figure of Latin American eugenics, was also ill and therefore absent; his place was

13. Ramos to Davenport, September 12, 1922, ibid.
14. Davenport to Ramos, November 9, 1922, ibid.
15. See Ramos to Davenport, July 31, 1923, ibid. Ramos assured Davenport that the Pan American organization would remain subordinate to the International Commission of Eugenics, over which Davenport presided.
16. See *Eugenical News* 8(5) (1923–1924): 39.
17. The numbers of participants were swelled by visitors who were not official delegates. Interestingly, Brazil was not represented. Argentina, Mexico, Chile, Peru, and the United States were among the countries that sent delegates.

taken by his deputy, Ramos, who in fact had engineered the meeting with energy and tenacity in order to set out a truly Pan American agenda for eugenics which would regulate and internationalize the movement.

By the time the Pan American Conference opened in 1927, Davenport's influence over its proceedings was considerable. It was on Davenport's recommendation that immigration was made a centerpiece of the debates, with the idea that through a Pan American eugenics umbrella organization, migration in the Americas could be regulated along eugenic lines. The 1924 immigration law in the United States had made evident the eugenic aspects of immigration policy by introducing new racial quotas; the law had provoked considerable discussion internationally. The Pan American Conference of Eugenics also took place against a background of anti-Chinese agitation in Cuba. Laughlin had made it clear in a letter to Ramos that the United States would not set quotas for Latin American immigrants as long as the Latin American countries maintained a standard of eugenic selection for immigrants comparable to that of the United States.[18] Another issue Ramos thought Davenport might like to raise at the conference was sterilization of criminals and mental defectives, as well as prenuptial certificates for the general population.[19]

As might be expected, once the conference started it became clear that Ramos and the U.S. delegates had developed a program that went far beyond what the Latin Americans were prepared for. The delegates were official representatives of their governments and had no authority to pass resolutions without consultation back home. The delegates were under considerable constraint about what they could endorse in public and understandably took a cautious line on eugenics. In addition, as we have seen, everything about Latin American eugenics in the 1920s oriented itself differently from that of the United States: its "soft" hereditarianism versus Davenport's "hard" Mendelism; the varieties and ambiguities of its racial ideologies versus Davenport's intransigent racism; its anxiety over extremism in the area of human reproduction versus U.S. interventionism.

18. Laughlin to Ramos, September 23, 1927, Davenport Papers, Ramos files, file 1 [note 5].

19. Ramos to Davenport, September 9, 1927 (on the eve of the conference), ibid. In the same letter Ramos told Davenport that Dr. Fernández, when he was in the House of Representatives, had presented a bill on eugenic sterilization.

The outcome of the conference was therefore far from what Ramos intended. Instead of agreement, there was disagreement; and the Latin American view of eugenics, not Davenport's, predominated. From the point of view of Ramos and the U.S. eugenists', the first Pan American Conference of Eugenics and Homiculture must be accounted a failure.

This failure was most obvious in the debate and votes concerning the Code of Eugenics and Homiculture, an extraordinary document that Ramos had drawn up in advance with the help of Davenport and Laughlin. Its contents can only have come as a shock to many of the delegates when he presented it to the conference for discussion and approval.[20] The code opened with a call for each Pan American nation to establish national archives of eugenics and institutes of anthropology and homiculture. Chapter 2 proposed requiring all individuals, when necessary, to divulge their biological-eugenic conditions to their governments so that they could be classified as eugenically "good," "doubtful," or "bad"; the reproductive life of persons classified as either bad or doubtful would come under the supervision of eugenics authorities, and "irresponsible" individuals would have to submit themselves to isolation, segregation, or sterilization. Chapter 3, on immigration, called for the free migration only of those individuals classified as germinally good and somatically "responsible"; and it gave the right to each Pan American nation to control decisions about immigration and to prohibit the entry of the eugenically unfit (or of any would-be immigrant from any American nation that had not signed the Pan American Code). The code proposed further to give each nation the right to establish social measures it considered necessary to conserve its racial purity and the right to choose the races that entered and formed part of its population. Chapter 5 returned to the problem of eugenic reproduction and fitness in marriage. Here the most controversial suggestion was to grant governments the right to annul marriages on eugenic criteria—crime, madness, untreated syphilis, or alcoholism contracted after marriage being grounds for such action.[21]

In his talk prefacing the code, Ramos classified the white race as

20. For an account of the conference in Spanish and English, see *Actas de la Primera Conferencia Panamericana de Eugenesia y Homicultura de las Repúblicas Americanas* (Havana: República de Cuba, 1928).

21. Ibid., pp. 147–73. The last chapters of the code, on milk centers for babies, physical education, and the relation between eugenics and sanitation, were relatively uncontroversial.

superior, and said that Latin Americans needed to imitate the United States on the issue of immigration and race. In recognition of the fact that some of the delegates represented countries where several races were found together, he recommended a eugenic program for each race separately and took a strong stand against racial crossing.[22] Demonstrating the new influence of Mendelism, he justified his stand as reflecting the principle of "aristocratic" generation. He indicated that he wanted maximum limitation of births, preferably by sterilization, to reduce the numbers of the unfit.[23]

The debate that followed Ramos's opening presentation, and Davenport's presentation on race crossing on the third day, indicated that the other Latin American delegates were hardly inclined to follow Ramos's lead on the Pan American Code of Eugenics. They showed tremendous hesitation about voting into being anything so extreme. They wanted study, education, propaganda; they wanted to preserve the right of each of their own countries to determine any measures having to do with population, migration, and the exit and entry of peoples; but they wanted no program so sweeping and radical as the one put before them.

Their resistance was most clear-cut on the proposals relating to reproduction. Throughout the history of Latin American eugenics, the avoidance of a zoological-technical approach to reproduction was a consistent theme. The suggestion that the population of each country should be eugenically classified and the rights of individuals to reproduction be decided on eugenic grounds of fitness shocked many delegates. One Argentinian, Dr. Raúl Cibils Aguirre, said he found that chapter of the code altogether "frightful." In his opinion, at the present moment there was nothing more difficult or dangerous than physical classification. He agreed with the other Argentinian delegates that any committment by his government to such a proposal would be completely premature and could come only after serious study. Articles 7 and 8, on segregation and sterilization, he rejected altogether. The delegate from Costa Rica sided with Cibils Aguirre, saying that reproduction was a private right and that his government would never accept the proposal. Further debate resulted in the delegates deciding to put aside any further discussion on these points.[24]

22. Ibid., pp. 47–58.
23. Ibid.
24. Ibid., pp. 101–3.

The reactions to the chapters of the code covering race and immigration were rather different. They reflected the evasions and sheer ambiguities of the racial theme within Latin American eugenics, especially in the face of the stridency of the Americans. On the one hand, as we have seen, the question of race was never far from the Latin American eugenists' minds. Many of them shared the United States's view that the Anglo-Saxon race was "best." On the other hand, it was painful to be told bluntly by others that Latin American nations were not eugenic. After all, was not the supposedly superior "Saxon race" (as Rafael Martínez Ortiz, Cuba's secretary of state, called it in his address of welcome) often in short supply in Latin America? Was not the racial crossing Ortiz and Davenport criticized commonplace in many countries?[25] And were not the immigration selection laws in the United States sometimes applied to Latin Americans in a negative and humiliating fashion? The Mexican delegate to the conference, Rafael Santamarina, for instance, felt called upon to defend the Indians from the charge of inferiority and to protest against the immigration tests the United States applied to Mexican children.[26]

But by far the strongest public opponent of the code's racist tone and policies was the Peruvian delegate, Dr. Carlos Enrique Paz Soldán, who for ten years or more had written on the need for a new "social medicine" and who was more and more finding himself involved with racial biology.[27] Paz Soldán's position at the conference seems somewhat surprising at first glance, because of his later view that Peru's ethnic identity was so fragile as to necessitate some kind of exclusion of "foreign" races, especially the Japanese, the bugbear of so many Peruvian intellectuals in the 1930s. Nevertheless, in 1927 something propelled him to oppose Ramos and the entire thrust of the code's racial proposals. Pride was one factor—underneath the fairly polite discourse, one senses a real irritation that the United States was trying to dictate policies that were not necessarily in the

25. See ibid., pp. 33–37, where Ortiz defined the Latin American stock as made up of two races—Anglo-Saxon and Latin. This definition was particularly narrow and racist coming from a Cuban, since the black population in Cuba was difficult to ignore.

26. Ibid., p. 72.

27. Marcos Cueto, "La historia de la ciencia y la tecnología en el Perú: Una aproximación bibliográfico," *Quipu: Revista Latinoamericana de la Historia de las Ciencias y la Tecnología* 4 (January–April 1987): 119–47, gives the references to the many writings of this Peruvian physician.

Latin Americans' best interests. It might be all very well for the Cubans, who were so much under the control of the United States, politically and financially, to adhere to the U.S. line on eugenics; but the delegates from the other Latin countries obviously felt rather differently.

Paz Soldán's argument was that the code was a "fantasy" unconnected to the racial realities of the area. He maintained that the language of race used in the code was confusing and imprecise, since most Latin Americans—Peruvians, Cubans, Argentinians, Chileans—did not yet form definite "races." He also found the suggestions about race control and immigration extraordinary from the point of view of practicality. Even with the best intentions, he said, legislation on the matter would "resuscitate the racial spirit, and would bring the most grave consequence of all—imperialism, political conflict, and inflammatory struggles."[28]

Ramos responded that if Latin Americans did not take action on immigration, the United States would, by setting eugenic or other quotas for Latin Americans trying to enter the United States. At this point Paz Soldán interrupted to remind Ramos and others that what made the United States great was precisely that so many different races lived there; but he also maintained that the issues of race were very complex and that one could not move easily beyond biological theory to policies without falling into sectarianism. The U.S. restriction on immigration might have a political or economic basis, he said, but it did not have a biological one.

Paz Soldán did not necessarily speak for all the Latin American delegates on the racial theme, but it was evident he expressed for many of them a worry about the way Davenport and Ramos had made the control of migration a purely racial issue. At the same time, on the grounds of national sovereignty, the delegates did not want to concede questions of the control of migration to any other country or organization. As a consequence they were inclined to keep some mention of the control of migration in the code.

The outcome was therefore a compromise. As a report on the Pan American Conference of Eugenics in the U.S. newsletter *Eugenical News* put it, the code Ramos proposed "was too mandatory and all

28. *Actas de la Primera Conferencia* [note 20], pp. 81–85. For anti-Japanese sentiment see *Primera Jornada Peruana de Eugenesia* (Lima, 1940); see also Carlos A. Bambarén, "La eugenesia en América," *Eugenesia* new ser. 1 (March 1940): 7–10.

mandatory statements were changed to recommendations or invitations."[29] The substance was also changed considerably. Gone were all references to direct reproductive-eugenic interventions, such as sterilization (the most sensitive issue within Latin American eugenics); the proposal to make prenuptial examinations for marriage compulsory was, however, kept.

On racial issues, the code that was approved indicated the ambivalent positions of the Latin American delegates, positions that included a commitment to some kind of "racial" component in eugenics and yet a resistance to a strong statement that might exacerbate the relations between Latin American countries. The code voted on gave each nation within the Pan American Union the right to form its own laws to prevent the entry of representatives of races it considered "undesirable," but it did not specifically mention eugenic and racial classification. The wording and the vote on the resolution no doubt reflected the Latins' deep desire for national autonomy in relation to their powerful neighbor to the north. In any event, none of the votes was binding on the national governments; the eugenic code was merely preliminary to further discussions and consultations.

The "Latinization" of Pan American Eugenics

Despite the disagreements that marked the First Pan American Conference of Eugenics, plans went forward for a second, to be held in Buenos Aires in 1930. Various factors caused the conference to be delayed until 1934. This delay was significant, because in the intervening period the international eugenics situation changed considerably.

First, in 1932 the United States hosted the Third International Congress of Eugenics. The meetings were dominated by the more extreme eugenists, and attention focused on problems of racial hybridization and international controls on immigration. But the extremism of the American eugenists was beginning, finally, to cause some embarrassment to the more sensible geneticists. The crass racist and class biases and the simple-minded, reductive genetics of Davenport and others had long caused unease, and several of the better-known geneticists had resigned from the American Breeders

29. *Eugenical News* 13 (February 1928): 17–19.

Association, the organization that had served as the national organization of eugenics. On the whole, disapproval and disagreement were kept private and quiet; many scientists believed that a public dispute would politicize science in a way that could only damage it. By hewing to a doctrine of scientific neutrality, these scientists made it difficult for others to attack the racism endemic in so much science at the time and deterred their own acknowledgment of the inherently political and social nature of the sciences of human variation. A few geneticists were more outspoken. In 1932, the geneticist Hermann J. Muller, for example, while he was at the Third International Congress of Eugenics, publicly derided eugenists for their simple-minded and prejudiced views (though he remained an advocate of a socialist eugenics).

The next year, in 1933, the National Socialists took power in Germany. Within a few months, the Nazis had passed the most sweeping eugenic legislation in existence.[30] Some eugenists in Europe and the United States greeted the legislation with interest and expectation, taking it for the boldest experiment in eugenics yet, but one that in many respects merely put into practice what the eugenists had long been preaching.[31] They saw it as the logical outcome of hereditary science and social needs. Other eugenists, on the contrary, were alarmed by the German sterilization law, especially as news of human rights abuses began to be received. There was a felt need, therefore, for a reassessment of eugenics among the more liberal scientists. In Britain, for instance, though a few members of the Eugenics Education Society followed the Nazis' lead and embraced fascism, most did not; instead they took pains to distance themselves from the Nazis while nevertheless keeping a eugenic identity that was faithful to its Mendelian roots.

Meanwhile, in Latin America, between the first and the second Pan American eugenics conferences, interest in eugenics had grown considerably. New societies had formed and political discussion had widened. The racial-reproductive themes within Latin American eugenics had been clarified. The changes in the national and interna-

30. Allan Chase, *The Legacy of Malthus* (Urbana: University of Illinois Press, 1980), pp. 133–35, points out that Laughlin's "model law," drawn up in 1922, served as a partial guide in the Nazi legislation.

31. See Donald E. McKenzie, *Statistics in Britain, 1865–1930: The Social Construction of Scientific Knowledge* (Edinburgh: Edinburgh University Press, 1981), pp. 44–45.

tional politics of eugenics, and the problematic relations between the Davenport-Laughlin wing and the Latin Americans made the Pan American eugenics meeting in Buenos Aires in 1934 even more complicated than the meeting of 1927. As in the earlier conference, but this time even more decisively, the Latin Americans rejected the U.S. agenda as unacceptable. The outcome was clearly to establish the predominance of a Latin point of view—both as to what eugenics was not and as to what it was. The ascendancy of the Latin tradition over that of the United States signaled, in effect, the end of the Pan American eugenics venture.

The Second Pan American Conference of Eugenics and Homiculture was slightly larger than the previous conference, having thirty-seven official delegates (compared to twenty-eight at the first). The conference was also more visible, because it was held in conjunction with the Pan American Sanitary Conference, which brought a large number of public-health officials, sanitarians, physicians, and demographers to Buenos Aires. It was no doubt in recognition of the international dimension of the conference that the meetings were opened in the presence of the president of the Argentine Republic, Agustín Justo. The occasion of the Pan American Sanitary Conference also allowed several of the smaller countries of Latin America—Haiti, Costa Rica, El Salvador, Honduras, Nicaragua, Panama—to send representatives to the eugenics conference.

As the host country, Argentina had a large stake in the conference's outcome. The Association of Biotypology, Eugenics, and Social Medicine provided the official delegates to the conference, and it was under some pressure to prevent the endorsement of reproduction guidelines that would offend public sensibilities. Davenport himself did not participate, as Ramos had hoped he would, though three others from the United States attended. On the other hand, Ramos faithfully represented Davenport's views to the conference members and in general acted as spokesman for the more extreme position within eugenics.

The "problem" of the conference became clear right at the beginning, in the opening address of the Argentine minister of external affairs, when, in welcoming the delegates to the city, he defined eugenics in terms of public health and sanitation. He even referred to the control of insect vectors that transmitted disease as a eugenic issue.[32] The minister's confusion about eugenics could perhaps have been excused on the grounds of ignorance, but that explanation could hardly have applied to several other Latin Americans who, in resisting the extreme positions put forward by Domingo y Ramos, insisted on placing eugenics within the broad spectrum of preventive medicine.

In this respect, the Uruguayans' presentation can serve as paradigmatic of the Latin approach. The Uruguayans had come armed with a new piece of social legislation, the Código del Niño (Children's Code), which exemplified their view of eugenics. The endorsement of this code, in fact, was one of the most symbolic acts of the conference.

The Uruguayans opened their presentation by reviewing, as they had been asked to do, the various eugenic initiatives undertaken in their country. They began with social welfare measures, which included aid to large families, the protection of abandoned infants, and the provision of homes for the indigent. This approach to eugenics contrasted with that of the U.S. members, who explicitly excluded sanitation and social welfare issues.[33] In discussing their country's initiatives in the sphere of reproduction, the Uruguayans pointed to the setting up of some marriage-counseling centers. Dr. Roberto Berro, the Uruguayan spokesman, indicated that these centers were governed by a set of "eugenic principles"—first, that eugenics was to be offered as "advice" and in as "broad and complete a form" as possible; and second, that any hygienic reproductive measures were to be entirely voluntary on the part of the individual concerned. There could be no imposition or obligation, only counsel and education.

Lastly, Dr. Berro turned to the *definition* of eugenics with which he operated. He did not believe, he said, that eugenics should limit itself to matters of heredity. To restrict eugenics in such a fashion would be to act like a farmer who buys the best seeds and then pays no attention to the way they develop. Since the study of heredity was very difficult, and since the eugenists had some ability to pre-

32. *Actas de la Segunda Conferencia Panamericana de Eugenesia y Homicultura de las Repúblicas Americanas* (Buenos Aires: Frascoli y Bindi, 1934), address by the minister of external relations and culture, Carlos Saavedra Lamas, pp. 18–21.

33. The Uruguayan presentation is found in ibid., pp. 48–51. A reference to the U.S. delegates' deliberate exclusion of social welfare issues is found on pp. 51–59.

pare the environment in which the child, well or badly born, could develop well, to linger too long on hereditary matters and fail to address the social powers now in the eugenists' hands would be to fail to achieve what everyone wanted, a "legitimate and logical" eugenics.[34]

To represent this enlarged vision of the "eugenic," the Uruguayans put forward for commendation, and they hoped emulation, their Código del Niño. This piece of legislation, passed in Uruguay just a few months before the conference, embraced all that the Uruguayans believed eugenics should be—a broad, noncoercive public-health and social welfare approach directed toward the child. Although the code made a space for hereditary issues and the "right of the child to be wellborn," it was predicated on the assumption that not all human characteristics were hereditary. This view required a reorientation of eugenics within the ecology of medical knowledge and practice.

On each of these points the majority of delegates followed the Uruguayans' lead. (Since the U.S. delegates were completely outvoted, and since only majority votes on the various proposals were recorded, one can understand why they tried to get the system changed to record votes country by country.) Agreeing to protect children was politically easy. Taking a united eugenic stand on reproduction was not. On this issue the Latins spoke almost with one voice. Moderation was the only route. Above all, sterilization was not to be thought of. To many delegates, eugenic sterilization was a zoological mutilation that lacked scientific rationale or moral sanction. Trying to salvage what he could from the situation, Ramos pressed for a consideration of at least voluntary sterilization. But the delegates would have none of it—they refused even to consider putting the issue to a vote.

In the wake of the papal encyclical of 1930, the Latin Americans had become so cautious, at least in public, on the issue of eugenic interference with reproduction that even prenuptial certificates were reexamined. The delegates therefore reversed their position of 1927 and endorsed only voluntary measures, a position that put them squarely within the official Catholic camp on the matter. This reversal of opinion was as much practical as moral. Paz Soldán pointed

34. Many of these ideas were becoming part of "reform" eugenics in Britain and the United States as well. On this point, see Kevles, *In the Name of Eugenics* [note 1], esp. chap. 11.

out that in Peru the attempt to mandate certificates had proved a failure. The certificates were easily purchased illegally or otherwise by-passed by the rich, and the poor either could not pay for them or would not take the trouble. (The matter continued to be debated right through the 1930s; as we have seen, many countries in Latin America did in fact mandate prenuptial tests.)

The disagreements between the "Anglo-Saxon" and the "Latin" views of the definition of eugenics were also interesting in other ways. Whereas the U.S. eugenists deliberately excluded public-health and social welfare measures from consideration, the Latin American delegates insisted on linking their eugenics to homiculture, as the Uruguayan delegation had done. Homiculture was, after all, what Ramos had first proposed as the region's original contribution to the field of eugenics. So persistent was the wider definition of eugenics that Ramos himself finally conceded the point, acknowledging that though he had planned the conference around only "eugenic" themes, he concluded that the Argentine and Uruguayan obstetricians and pediatricians would not confine themselves in that way.[35] Far from failing, then, the Second Pan American Conference of Eugenics and Homiculture perhaps succeeded in living up to its name.

In this regard, the role of Paz Soldán at the second conference was as critical as it had been at the first. It also demonstrated that resistance to U.S. power in the sphere of science could be very complicated. Paz Soldán's contribution to the issue came as a direct response to Domingo y Ramos's reading of the paper Laughlin prepared for the conference on the topic of race in the Americas. As we know, the issue of race was never far away when the Latin Americans discussed eugenics. In the 1930s, as we have seen too, several countries had begun to put in place their own controls over immigration, partly, it is true, on economic grounds, but also on "eugenic" ones.

Yet the Latin American delegates were not always comfortable with the United States's insistence on identifying eugenics with the racial theme and were always sensitive to their own racial identities when they were viewed negatively from the outside. This discomfort, especially in a public conference that included delegates from several Latin American countries that were clearly not white, was indicated once again by Paz Soldán's refusal to follow the lead of

35. *Actas de la Segunda Conferencia Panamericana de Eugenesia* [note 32], p. 154.

Ramos in eugenics, on the grounds that the exclusive focus on racial eugenics did an injustice to the population problems in the region. Paz Soldán's opposition was especially important because, unlike some of the other delegates, he was quite comfortable about reserving the term "eugenics" for heredity and heredity alone. On the other hand, Paz Soldán was damned if U.S. eugenics, with its racism and its views on sterilization, was going to monopolize what he himself had defined, as long ago as 1916, as the new "social medicine." Eugenics by itself, said Paz Soldán, could not be the lynchpin of modern medicine, because to make it so would be to sever the norms established in sanitation and to focus attention on a very small part indeed of what affected the health and vitality of populations. Thus though he acknowledged the importance of "eugenics" as the U.S. group understood it, he was at one with the other Latin Americans in thinking that eugenics was very far from encompassing the whole truth about health.

The rather refined sense of eugenics, social medicine, and race came out most clearly in Paz Soldán's resistance to Ramos's plea for a study of the eugenic-racial health of Latin America along the racial lines set forth by Laughlin. Paz Soldán insisted that there was much more to the population problem in Latin America than race. Disease, labor conditions, and exploitation all determined the health of populations. To study them along eugenic lines alone would be to narrow the inquiry. Paz Soldán then posited the work of a fellow Peruvian, Dr. Carlos Monge, pioneer in the scientific study of high-altitude physiology among the Indians, as an example not of narrow "eugenics," but of broad-gauged "social medicine."[36]

This was no simple battle over terminology—eugenics versus social medicine. Nor was it a battle simply over Lamarckian versus Mendelian visions of how heredity worked. Paz Soldán and many other delegates were refusing to confine their attention, even at a conference ostensibly about eugenics, to the field of heredity and selection as Ramos and Laughlin defined it, especially a eugenics burdened by a severe racial ideology and by stringent reproductive policies.

36. On Monge, see Marcos Cueto, "Andean Biology in Peru: Scientific Styles on the Periphery," *Isis* 80 (1989): 640–58.

The Latin International Federation of Eugenics Societies

Even before the Second Pan American Conference of Eugenics and Homiculture met in Buenos Aires in 1934, the Latins had begun to reach out for a new international organization that would express better than the existing ones their special sense of Latinity and eugenics. This was the Latin International Federation of Eugenics Societies (Federación Internacional Latina de Sociedades de Eugenesia), apparently proposed first by the veteran Italian eugenist and past president of the Italian Society of Genetics and Eugenics, Dr. Corrado Gini, as a way of representing what he called certain "Latin commonalities."

By 1933 preparatory meetings for such an organization had already been held, and by 1934 the statutes had been drawn up.[37] In 1935, a preliminary, and primarily organizational session was held in Mexico City.[38] Delegates from Argentina, Peru, and Mexico, with the support of eugenics societies in Brazil, Belgium, France, and Italy and the participation of interested parties from Colombia, Cuba, Costa Rica, Uruguay, Honduras, Panama, and elsewhere, agreed to encourage the formation of eugenics societies in all the Latin countries and to hold their first official congress in Paris in 1937.[39]

Given the broad scope of its Latin membership, it is interesting to know what Gini meant by the "commonalities" that supposedly bound the diverse countries and eugenic activities together. What stands out is that "Latinity" was constructed as an oppositional identity to "Anglo-Saxonism." The latter was taken to stand for dogmatic interpretation, hasty action in application, and too rigid an identification of eugenics with narrow hereditarianism. The former

37. The preparatory meeting was reported in the *Anales de Biotipología, Eugenesia y Medicina Social* 1 (April 15, 1933): 11. The statutes were reported in the Mexican journal *Eugenesia* 2 (March 30, 1934): 1.

38. See *Anales de Biotipología, Eugenesia y Medicina Social* 3 (December 1, 1935): 23. Another report appeared in the French *Revue Anthropologique* (which published the work of the French Eugenics Society) 46 (1936): 190–91.

39. Also agreeing to be associated with the new federation were the eugenics societies of Catalonia (Spain), Portugal, Rumania, and Switzerland. The conference was scheduled for just before or immediately after the international congress of anthropology to be held in Bucharest that year.

was taken to mean moderation in interpretation, caution in application, and a more ample sense of the sphere of social action. Latinity really meant opposition to an intervenionist reproductive eugenics.

The Latin federation also claimed another area of differentiation, namely race. The Anglo-Saxon view was seen as one-sided and excessively biological; the Latin was claimed to be multiple, reflecting the diversities of the Latin American racial situation, as well as spiritual or philosophical, the result of a more tolerant view of race. Of course, as we have seen in the analysis of Argentine eugenics in the 1930s, such notions of Latinity, many of them reflecting Italian Fascist notions hardly compatible with the black and mulatto elements of many countries of Latin America, incorporated its own forms of racism, whatever the language used to express it. A Latin sense of race did not prevent debate on the themes of race crossing and immigration at the first official congress of the federation. Nevertheless, the Latin International Federation of Eugenics Societies, in setting itself up in contradistinction to other international eugenics organizations, claimed to draw on an older pedigree of Latin identity in eugenics, based on the feeling that the variety of populations that made up Latin countries, the "moderation" of Latin culture, even its "detachment," rendered a Latin perspective on eugenics unique.

In 1936 Corrado Gini, serving as president of the new organization, articulated this tradition in the Argentine *Annals of Biotypology, Eugenics, and Social Medicine*.[40] Gini stressed two themes: the diversity of the populations the new Latin federation represented and the commitment to restraint in applying principles. The very diversity of the Latin American countries, in short, gave them their commonalities. Some countries in the area were immigrant, others not; some had high birth rates, others low; some countries felt that their national identity was threatened by population currents coming in from the outside, while others welcomed such currents. All these variations signified the inability of eugenics to stand for unilateral and dogmatic positions and made Latin America, Gini claimed, the setting for objectivity and impartiality. Latin America was like a vast laboratory of peoples, races, and health, in which human beings

40. Corrado Gini, "Vecchi problemi e nuovi indirizzi nel campo dell'eugenica," *Anales de Biotipología, Eugenesia y Medicina Social* 3 (May 1, 1936): 5–6.

could not be considered merely animals whose rights could be subordinated to a collective interest.

In 1932 the Argentines had asked themselves what was left of eugenics given uncertainty about the laws of heredity and moral restraints on social legislation; now Gini asked the same question and gave the same answer. On the issue of uncertainty, he evoked the names of the U.S. geneticists William Castle, Thomas Hunt Morgan, Herbert Jennings, and Raymond Pearl, all of whom had criticized eugenists for their simple-minded notions of inheritance. But whereas some people had concluded from these criticisms that eugenics was therefore useless, to Gini what collapsed was not eugenics in its entirety "but only the specific ideas of groups of eugenists." And in the now familiar and almost classic formulation of Latin eugenics, he spoke of the need not for positive or negative eugenics but for a "renovative" eugenics.[41]

But the time for expressing that sense of Latinity in eugenics was about to pass. The extreme positions taken by some U.S. eugenicists, which had alienated many of their colleagues in the United States as well as in France and Latin America, was followed by the extreme racism of Nazi eugenics. This extremism forced a reassessment of eugenics in its entirety. Support for *any* kind of eugenics was, in effect, disappearing. The Nuremberg laws of the Third Reich, prohibiting marriages between Gentiles and Jews, had been put into effect in 1935, and their insidious meaning, as well as their intertwining with the Nazi eugenic legislation of 1933, was beginning to be understood. The Nazi developments prompted the head of the French Anthropological Society, in whose facilities the French Eugenics Society held its meetings, to try to close the Eugenics Society in 1936. William H. Schneider concludes that when the first congress of the Latin International Federation of Eugenics Societies was held in Paris in 1937, support for even a "mild" eugenics—one that reflected, as the incoming president of the Latin federation, Eugène Apert, put it, their "older and more moderate" Latin culture—had evaporated.[42] The claim that the Latins' biological-hereditary eu-

41. This brought Latin eugenics close to what Kevles has called "reform eugenics"; see Kevles, *In the Name of Eugenics* [note 1], chap. 11.

42. William Schneider, "Eugenics in France," in *The Wellborn Science: Eugenics in Germany, France, Brazil, and Russia*, ed. Mark B. Adams (New York: Oxford University Press, 1990), pp. 69–109.

genics movement was unlike the others, or had nothing to do with racism, was now shown to be empty. In any event, only Renato Kehl from Brazil contributed a paper, and not in person. In this sense, the Congress was hardly a Latin American affair. It was, in effect, the last gasp of a French tradition of eugenics, before the defeat of France by Germany opened the doors to Nazi-style racial policies.[43]

The Decline of Eugenics?

For anyone writing the history of eugenics, the problem of continuities and discontinuities in the 1930s is of fundamental interpretive significance. This is especially true of German eugenics, for the obvious reason that eugenics under the Nazis was pushed to such awful and malignant extremes that one has to question whether the German tradition in eugenics before 1933, dating back to at least 1905 if not earlier, can itself explain the extremity of eugenics under the Nazis after 1933. Or was there something fundamentally different about the racial eugenics of the Nazis, especially its extreme anti-Semitism?[44] These questions are, of course, part of the larger and extraordinarily difficult problem of how to explain the Nazis, and especially the Holocaust, in German history.

In other extreme eugenics movements the question of continuity and discontinuity is also important. Kevles takes the view that in the 1930s in the United States, a "reform" eugenics came into being that was purged of its earlier racism, classism, and extremism. He argues that the fortunes of what he calls "mainline" eugenics declined with

43. The congress produced a report, published as Fédération International Latine des Sociétés d'Eugénique, I Congrès Latin d'Eugénique, *Rapport* (Paris, 1937). Renato Kehl's paper was printed as "Valeur comparée de l'acroissement qualitatif et quantitatif d'une population (Résultat d'une enquête faite avec 500 couples)," pp. 73–78.

44. This issue is far from being settled. To answer it requires more detailed studies of the continuities in themes and personnel within eugenics and medicine and of the discontinuities in policies after 1933. For instance, the sexual radicalism with which eugenics was associated before 1933 came to an abrupt end that year; birth-control clinics were closed, sex-education courses prohibited, antiabortion laws strictly imposed. Nazi eugenics was highly class-, gender-, and race-specific, in ways that also broke continuities. On these issues see Sheila Faith Weiss, "The Race Hygiene Movement in Germany," *Osiris* 2d ser. 3 (1987): 193–236, and her chapter on German eugenics in *The Wellborn Science* [note 42], pp. 8–68.

the drive for eugenic sterilization. For instance, attendance at the Third International Congress of Eugenics in New York in 1932 was much lower than at the previous congress of 1921. In 1935 the Carnegie Institution, which funded the Eugenics Record Office, was ready to withdraw its support of eugenics research; in 1939 Laughlin was finally persuaded to retire, and in 1940 the office itself was closed. Interest in eugenics did not, however, disappear; out of the decline of the older eugenics associated with explicit racism, flawed and simplistic science, and extreme social measures there emerged a new or reformulated eugenics. Eventually the scientific field that eugenics had encompassed was reconstituted as the new field of "human genetics," ostensibly a neutral field of knowledge without the ideological underpinnings of the previous era. According to this interpretation, reform eugenics was more "scientific" as well as more liberal and/or progressive, and as such was espoused by liberal scientists such as the British J. B. S. Haldane, Lancelot Hogben, and Julian Huxley. Kevles, then, stresses a certain "rupture" and "reconstruction" of eugenics in the late 1930s and 1940s, under the pressure of changes in science and politics.[45]

Other historians see the situation differently. Garland Allen, for instance, acknowledges a gradual metamorphosis of eugenics and genetics in the 1930s and 1940s, especially in reaction to Nazi eugenics, but argues that these changes involved only the outer structure and left the core beliefs and their associated social structures (race, class) intact. He emphasizes the resilience of eugenics and the continuities in its history; he sees its old commitment to hereditary and racial control remaining in new guises. Even though eugenics became a dirty word, its ideas persisted within the restructured field of human genetics which emerged after World War II.[46] Others, too, would question whether the new field of human genetics escaped the value conflicts and implicit political projects of society—whether one *can* separate science from ideology.

Several Latin countries of Europe as well as Latin America had, as we have seen, long thought of their eugenics as scientifically and socially set apart from that of the Anglo-Saxons. News of the Nazi policies in eugenics reached Latin America, but disapproval of Nazi

45. See Kevles, *In the Name of Eugenics* [note 1], chap. 11.
46. Garland Allen, "From Eugenics to Population Control: The Work of Raymond Pearl," *Science for the People*, July/August 1980, pp. 22–28.

reproductive policy at least was already strongly expressed. The very lateness of eugenics in Latin America and the unselfconscious way eugenics continued to be endorsed, if in a vague fashion, right into the 1940s and later, testify to the distance Latin American eugenists could profess to feel from what was going on in Nazi Germany.

Many of the eugenics societies or organizations persisted, even into the 1940s, as they did in so many other countries in Europe, including Britain.[47] It is true that a decision was made to replace the Third Pan American Conference of Eugenics, planned to be held in Colombia in 1938, with a Congress of Puericulture; this shift indicated a return to the puericulture roots of Latin eugenics and a conscious desire to move away from the word "eugenics." But in many cases, a process of deliberate retreat from extremism was not seen to be necessary. Also noticeable was the continued expectation of the promise of eugenics in the future.

Even the commitment to neo-Lamarckism proved remarkably long-lasting. The surprise the Russian-born, American-based geneticist Theodosius Dobzhansky felt at finding so many Brazilian biologists still committed to neo-Lamarckian notions in the early 1940s has been mentioned earlier.[48] Dobzhansky made several research visits to Latin America and played a part in stimulating the development of modern, experimental genetics in several institutions. In Mexico, José Rulfo was introducing Mendelian genetics in his biology courses by the early 1940s; even before that, the eugenist Alfredo Saavedra, in his short textbook, *Notions of Biology* (1939), repudiated the notion of the inheritance of acquired characteristics.

Nevertheless, one can find traces of lingering Lamarckism in

47. In 1942 the Mexican Eugenics Society, according to José Rulfo, had 112 members and was trying to get government support for a department of eugenics. As late as 1950, Enrique Días de Guijarro was calling himself the vice president of the Argentine Society of Eugenics. See his "Libertad, moral y amor: Problemas jurídicos de la eugenesia," *Pediatría de las Américas* 8 (January 1950): 124–25.

48. Dobzhansky's interaction with Mexican geneticists is also interesting. In 1938 Dobzhansky visited Mexico, where he engaged in a dialogue with the zoologist Enrique Beltrán about the "dialectical materialism" espoused by the French biologist and Communist party member Marcel Prenant. Beltrán was very taken with Prenant's work, which he translated into Spanish; Beltrán also produced a book of his own on the topic. Nevertheless, Beltrán formed a firm friendship with Dobzhansky and eventually endorsed his strict Mendelism and neo-Darwinism. See Enrique Beltrán, "Theodosius Dobzhansky," *Revista de la Sociedad Mexicana de Historia Natural* 37 (December 1976): 43–49.

Mexican biology well into the 1940s.[49] Even in Argentina, in so many respects the most industrially advanced and richest of the Latin American countries, neo-Lamarckian ideas remained until late, hidden, it is true, in Mendelian language. As José Andrés, professor of genetics and plant technics at the University of Buenos Aires, remarked in his textbook of 1943, "We have incorporated genetics a little slowly in our country."[50] The appearance of Herbert Jennings's *Biological Bases of Human Behavior* in a Spanish-language edition in 1942 (it had first appeared in English in 1930) revealed many biological fallacies that were of great use to Latin Americans, especially to doctors, and especially those fallacies concerning the inheritance of acquired characteristics. Yet there remained a deep-seated conviction that such things as alcohol abuse could permanently affect human chromosomes.[51]

Eugenics, therefore, suffered no sudden rupture in Latin America. It remained true to its type, though its advocates diminished in numbers. What did finally come about was a convenient disclaimer that the Latin Americans had ever espoused eugenic principles. Convenient because, by the time the war had ended, the Nazis' forcible sterilization of more than 350,000 people in the name of eugenics and their extermination of millions of Jews in the name of "race inferiority" had caused such profound revulsion that the very word "eugenics" became taboo.

No wonder, then, that the Latin Americans found it easiest to say they had never indulged in the madness that had swept the more extreme Anglo-Saxon countries. They thus forgot their own involvement, albeit on their own terms and in their own fashion, with a scientistic movement of dubious value but of international scope.

49. See, e.g., Federico Pascual del Roncal, "Fundamentos biológicos de la herencia," *Eugenesia* new ser. 2 (November 30, 1941): 4–13, where the author reviewed the work of Mendel, Weismann, and Morgan, and the debate on the inheritance of acquired characteristics. He said that while most biologists rejected the notion of the inheritance of acquired characteristics and that experimental evidence in its favor was lacking, nevertheless he believed that certain abnormal experiences in the intra-uterine period could have effects on the "germinal genes."

50. José Andrés, *La herencia en el hombre: Anomalías y enfermedades* (Buenos Aires: Ateneo, 1943), p. 7. It is interesting to note that Andrés, in adopting the Mendelian position, also endorsed sterilization as it was practiced in the United States and northern Europe (p. 74).

51. On this point, see, for instance, Juan Pou Orfila, "Reflexiones sobre la eugénica en América Latina," *Obstétrica y Ginecología Latino-Americana* 5(1) (1943): 50–65.

7
Conclusion: Science and the Politics of Interpretation

In this book, I have emphasized the role of eugenics in representation, especially the representation of race, gender, and nationality. I have stressed thereby the "ideological work" of eugenics, meaning by ideology a normal and inescapable part of all discourses and social practices. As Mary Poovey (from whom I have taken the expression "ideological work") has argued in her study of Victorian fiction, ideology should be thought of not as an extra or "biased" aspect of life which, once identified, can be removed as "false," but as a routine, everyday product of social relations and lived experiences.[1] Science is different from fiction in its discursive structures and forms, but it too grows out of, and is connected to, the social life of individuals and groups in multiple and changing ways. Scientists are part of the society in which they live, and as men and women, members of particular social classes, participants in religious and social organizations, members of households, they participate in the values and politics of their times.

Their scientific representations are therefore shaped by, as well as shape, the world around them. This constitutive and representative

1. Mary Poovey's *Uneven Developments: The Ideological Work of Gender in Mid-Victorian England* (Chicago: University of Chicago Press, 1988). A discussion of ideology also appears in her first book, *The Proper Lady and the Woman Writer* (Chicago: University of Chicago Press, 1985), pp. xii–xiv.

work of science cannot, however, be reduced in any straightforward way to social and economic determinants. Although at times eugenics can certainly be said to have served certain class or economic interests, no simple social determinant explanation does justice to the varieties of attitudes and positions people held on eugenics. While nearly all eugenists belonged to the professional and/or middle class, so did their opponents. Eugenics appealed to people on the left as well as the right; attracted some women but was also directed against them; was endorsed by mulatto professionals such as Juliano Moreira in Brazil but was also used against all members of "lower races" by others. In every case we look at, eugenics was embedded in local value systems and connected to larger, even international systems of communication and value, and the meanings and social uses of eugenics cannot be understood without reference to these various contexts.

The history of eugenics in Latin America shows that even the adoption of a specific scientific theory within scientific circles and elsewhere is not a purely empirical, logical, or evidential matter but a historical and political one. Science is usually not uniform or monochrome, but full of diversity and even contradictions, so that aspects of science that get taken up by particular groups or attached to specific institutions cannot be explained solely by reference to their purely factual character or truth status, as though these were direct, unproblematic features of knowledge.

We have seen that neo-Lamarckian theories of heredity were widespread in Latin American medical and biological circles for a variety of cultural, structural, political, and intellectual reasons. The long-standing reliance on French definitions in science was one basis of the Latin Americans' emphasis on what later would be seen to be an unscientific theory of inheritance. After the rediscovery of Mendel's laws of inheritance (a rediscovery that was itself a result of social and political as well as intellectual and scientific factors), the field of genetics became defined in more precise, experimental terms. As a field, it also became more obviously contentious, so that the details of the theories of heredity employed by doctors and biologists became matters of more self-conscious appraisal. Lamarckism emerged in this context as neo-Lamarckism—as a particular scientific orientation toward problems of environmental-genetic interaction. In the circumstances, we can see how puericulture, a preexisting medical model for dealing with the apparent "depopulation" caused by high maternal death rates and infant mortality and morbidity, should begin to acquire a more specifically eugenic-hereditarian identity. A "soft" theory of heredity allowed a great deal of flexibility when it came to explaining human illness and suggesting practical policies of reform; politically, such a theory served the interests of doctors, since *qua* theory it legitimated a medical-interventionist approach to health.

Other features of the political culture in early twentieth-century Latin America played their parts in giving eugenics its resonance and its peculiar character. Here I would single out first the political visibility and ideological weight of the sanitation sciences and the managerial-technical approach to the health of human populations in many countries of the region. Puericulture-before-birth initially joined with, rather than stood against, sanitation; the eugenists sought allies in the field of public hygiene, so that professional rivalries between distinct groups were minimized. The result was that the two fields tended to merge. Second, the generally pronatalist bias of doctors, so noticeable in France at the end of the nineteenth century, in Latin America also tended initially to turn eugenics in a reformist "mother-child" direction. The desire for more people, and more healthy people, in Brazil, for example, where death rates of poor people were extraordinarily high and fertility and natural population growth among the working population therefore low, made the idea of a deliberate policy to reduce population in the name of health unacceptable to policy makers. In Mexico, the huge destruction of human life during the years of revolution made propopulation ideas a consistent theme in medical and political circles right through the 1920s and 1930s. In addition, in the countries studied here, traditional attitudes toward gender and the family restrained the majority of eugenists from putting forward such extreme eugenic proposals as sterilization. This mix of intellectual, cultural, economic, and political circumstances produced in the first instance an anti-Malthusian, neo-Lamarckian, social eugenics in many parts of Latin America.

Given British and U.S. definitions of eugenics, the eugenics of the Latin Americans perhaps seemed barely to meet the criteria of the new science and social movement. Yet as I have said, Latin America must be seen less as apart from the mainstream of eugenics than as within an alternative stream of eugenics. Natural selection, hard genetic theories, and extreme views took second place to environmental reforms and the elimination of so-called racial poisons because of the general feeling that such reforms would "improve the race."

As the political conditions in which science operates change, the political messages derived from it change too. In the 1930s Latin American eugenics shifted toward a more negative outlook on heredity, race, and gender. In this era prenuptial tests and certificates were mandated by law, immigration-restriction laws with eugenic elements were passed, and there was talk of making inventories of the nations' germ plasms. In the wake of the depression and new immigration laws in Europe and the United States, conservative ideologies proliferated, antiforeign feeling intensified, and racism grew more public in many areas of Latin America. Where there had once been a generalized, somewhat optimistic pronatalist outlook, there now developed within some eugenics movements a more selectively differentiated pronatalism. What had been originally an environmentally focused, even at times "progressive" movement turned toward harsher eugenic programs.

Thus the political messages extracted from science were variable. Similarly, one could analyze the intellectual, political, and other factors surrounding the ways in which Mendelism was taken up and given authority, and the various meanings that seemed "naturally" to follow from it. The case of Brazil shows, for instance, that the contrasting theory of "hard" heredity, which we usually associate with "hard" policies of eugenic segregation, sterilization, and a rejection of traditional sanitary reforms of the environment, could also provide the cognitive basis for a critical attitude toward this kind of eugenics. Mendelism was taken up in Brazil in the 1920s and 1930s because it was the theory adopted in the United States, to which young scientists were increasingly turning for their scientific training; because Mendelism provided, as neo-Lamarckism did not, specific experimental methods that could be employed in agriculture to improve productivity; and because of the influence of some key figures, such as Boas (and later Dobzhansky), who were critical of the racism and intellectual simplicities of eugenics as it was understood in the United States at the time. The turn to a more conservative eugenics in the 1930s did not, therefore, go uncontested by the new Mendelians.

These examples illustrate the varieties of social Lamarckism and social Mendelism that could exist in different political circumstances. They also show that science is never organized in a value-free environment but is given meaning and creates new meaning in settings that are specifically social, economic, and political as well as intellectual. This kind of claim, however, does not mean that science can be bent at will by political circumstances or that we should think of the genetics of the eugenists as only pseudoscience. First, at the time all the parties involved were seen as participating in normal scientific work. Unless we are ready to dismiss all of genetics and eugenics between 1900 and 1930 as a pseudoscience, we have to be able to examine the intermingling of scientific, social, and political values as a routine and usual part of scientific work. Second, there were limits to the kinds of policies or conclusions that could be derived from a science of heredity. Genetics in the early twentieth century was a new way of organizing people's understanding of how to think of variation in animal and plant populations, what the environment did to that variation, and how human agency could, as a consequence, manipulate aspects of human variation. Hereditarianism was innovative conceptually and technically; it indicated certain lines of social action and not others. Within these lines, however, there was scope for interpretive maneuver, and it is the politics of these interpretations that I have pursued.

Something further needs to be said about the politics of eugenics (I use the word "politics" here in the more traditional sense of political party alignment). People still tend to associate eugenics automatically with conservative or reactionary (fascistic) politics. Some historians have been reluctant to accept the fact that in the 1920s, and even in the 1930s, eugenics was at times promoted by left-wing and socialist individuals and groups. Hermann J. Muller, who won the Nobel Prize for genetics (for his discovery in 1927 of X-ray induced genetic mutation), was a socialist who in the 1930s proselytized a scheme for genetic selection through the artificial insemination of women by the superior sperm of "great men." Kevles describes the great enthusiasm with which Muller's book *Out of the Night* was greeted when it appeared in Britain in 1936—it sold 13,000 copies through the Left Wing Book Club.[2] The case of Mexico is another

2. Daniel J. Kevles, *In the Name of Eugenics: Genetics and the Uses of Human Heredity* (New York: Knopf, 1987), p. 191. Kevles remarks on Muller's extraordinary attitude toward women: only men were involved in eugenic selection; he assumed that the quality of women's germ plasm was of little importance to the quality of the offspring. Muller also believed that any woman would be "proud to bear and rear a child of Lenin or of Darwin" (p. 191).

example; the fact that the state of Veracruz legislated (however briefly) involuntary sterilization for eugenic purposes reminds us that materialist, state-led, top-down, technocratic, secular approaches toward reproduction appealed to the left because they challenged the traditional, religious view of sexuality and reproduction and offered a modern, scientific approach to reproductive health. Eugenics on the left was very much the exception in Latin America. On the whole, the eugenists operated in a political, cultural, and religious climate in which birth control, abortion for any but the most strictly defined medical reasons, and sterilization, whether for eugenic or feminist purposes, were unacceptable. The eugenics movements tended to be associated with antifeminist ideas and liberal-to-conservative political parties. And in the 1930s many eugenists in Brazil and Argentina could probably best be called semifascist in political orientation.

One general conclusion to be drawn from this synopsis of the history of eugenics in Latin America between 1918 and 1940 is the need to avoid simple reductionism or essentialism in the history of science. As I mentioned in the Introduction, Thomas Glick has shown that studying the scientific reception of Darwin's theory of evolution by natural selection, Einstein's theory of relativity, or Freud's psychoanalysis in different countries raises interesting questions about what is to count as normative in science.[3] The history of eugenics in Latin America confirms his point: for much of the time eugenics was not the stereotypical hard-line, politically conservative, neo-Mendelian movement characteristic of eugenics in the United States and Germany in the late 1920s, but it was not for that reason to be counted out of eugenics.

The history of eugenics should alert us to the politics of scientific interpretation. As we enter a new stage in genetics, biotechnology, and reproductive physiology, we have to be constantly aware that our sciences, and the social messages we derive from them, are never "simply scientific" but are complex constructions that always involve struggles over meaning and values.

3. See especially Thomas F. Glick, "Cultural Issues in the Reception of Relativity," in *Comparative Reception of Relativity*, ed. Thomas F. Glick (Dordrecht: D. Reidel, 1987), pp. 381-400.

Index

Eugenics
Anglo-Saxon vs. Latin views of, 2–4,
85, 177–78, 182–88
decline of, 192–95
definition of, 1–2, 185
and evolution, 22–26, 41, 91
international aspects of, 18–19, 28,
171–72, 189–92 (*see also* Pan American eugenics, history of)
negative, 22, 30, 87-88, 102, 107-34,
150, 158-59 (*see also* Matrimonial
eugenics)
not unitary, 2–4
origins of, 35–46
political meanings of, 61–62
positive, 30, 87
preventive, 17-18, 85, 87, 100-101
(*see also* Puericulture, and eugenics;
Racial poisons)
reform, 186*n*, 191–93
social change and, 38–49, 100–101
in United States, 172
Eugenics Education Society (England),
28, 91, 108*n*, 171, 183
Eugenics Record Office (U.S.), 28,
172, 174*n*, 193
Eugenists, use of term, 1*n*
Euphrenia, 52
Evolution, 22–26, 68, 74. *See also* Social Darwinism

Family, and social policy, 43–44
Fascism, 163, 183. *See also* Italian fas-
cism; Nazi eugenics
Federación Internacional Latina de
Sociedades de Eugenesia. *See* Latin
International Federation of Eu-
genics Societies
Fernández, Ubaldo, 82
Fernández Verano, Alfredo, 82–83
"Ficha biotipológica," 119, 121
First Universal Races Congress (Lon-
don), 155
Fonseca, Froés de, 162
Fontanelle, Oscar, 127, 161
Forel, Auguste, 84
France
eugenics in, 80–81, 87, 138
Latin American medicine and, 72–79,
198
prenuptial testing and, 124, 127
French Eugenics Society, 28, 47, 80, 82

Freyre, Gilberto, 45, 160, 167–69
Frías, Jorge A., 91, 125

Gallardo, Angel, 70
Galton, Francis, 1, 22–26, 30, 83, 96
Gamio, Manuel, 147, 151
García de Mendoza, Adalberto, 73
Gemelli, Father Agostino, 118
Gender
differential constructions of, 127–28
and eugenics, 12, 17, 60, 103–4, 107–
11, 127–28
meaning of, 12–14
and race, 13–14, 18
and reproduction, 12
See also Women
Genetics
multiple meanings and, 17
relation to eugenics, 24–26, 86
See also Heredity; Lamarckism; Men-
delian genetics; Science
German Society for Race Hygiene, 28,
158
Germany
anti-Jewish policies in, 143–44
sex reform movement in, 108–9
See also Nazi eugenics
Gini, Corrado, 115, 189–91
Glick, Thomas F., 3, 201
Gobineau, Joseph Arthur, Count de,
45, 155
González, José Eduardo, 150*n*
Gould, Stephen Jay, 14*n*
Graham, Loren, 136
Great Britain, 39, 91, 183

Hahner, June E., 109
Harriman, Mrs. E. H., 172
Health. *See* Mental hygiene; Public
health; Racial poisons; Sanitation;
Venereal disease
Heath, Shirley Brice, 145, 150
Herbert, S., 111*n*
Hereditary Genius (Galton), 22–26
Heredity
and eugenics movement, 5, 22–27,
188
health and, 9, 24, 32
racial poisons and, 85–86, 100–101
sanitation and, 50, 84–85
See also Blastophthoria; Lamarckism;
Mendelian genetics
Hernández, Eusebio, 76, 78–79, 176